*Arterial
Surgery
of the
Lower Limb*

Published volume in this Series

Operative Paediatric Urology
J. David Frank and J. H. Johnston

PRACTICE OF SURGERY

Arterial Surgery of the Lower Limb

P. R. F. BELL MB CHB FRCS MD

Professor of Surgery,
University of Leicester

ILLUSTRATIONS BY
PATRICK ELLIOT
Medical Illustration Department,
Sheffield

Churchill Livingstone

EDINBURGH LONDON MELBOURNE AND NEW YORK 1991

CHURCHILL LIVINGSTONE
Medical Division of Longman Group UK Limited

Distributed in the United States of America by
Churchill Livingstone Inc., 1560 Broadway, New
York, N.Y. 10036, and by associated companies,
branches and representatives throughout the
world.

First published 1991

ISBN 0 443 03541 5

British Library Cataloguing in Publication Data

Bell, P. R. F. (Peter Robert Frank)
    Arterial surgery of the lower limb.
    1. Man. Legs. Veins. Surgery
    I. Title   II. Series
    617.584

**Library of Congress Cataloging in
Publication Data**

Bell, Peter R. F. (Peter Robert Frank)
    Arterial surgery of the lower limb/P.R.F. Bell; illustrations
  by Patrick Elliott.
        p.   cm.—(Practice of surgery)
    Includes index.
    ISBN 0-443-03541-5
    1. Arteries—Surgery.   2. Extemities, Lower—Blood-vessels—
  Surgery.   I. Title.   II. Series.
      [DNLM: 1. Arteries—surgery.   2. Leg—surgery.   WE 850 B434a]
    RD560.B45   1991
    617.4'13—dc20
    DNLM/DLC
    for Library of Congress   90-2320
                                                            CIP

Printed and bound in Great Britain by
William Clowes Limited, Beccles and London

Vascular surgery, above all else, is a speciality which demands technical excellence, especially when more distal procedures are being undertaken. The results of these procedures are said to vary widely but depend, I believe, on almost obsessional attention to detail. If done correctly, then a successful outcome will save the limb in many frail and elderly patients who would otherwise be bedridden by an amputation. If done incorrectly, however, then the unfortunate patient is exposed to unnecessary operations and a higher mortality. Quite apart from technical excellence, there are a number of other factors which will contribute to success or failure of a graft, including proper preoperative preparation and case selection. This short book aims to deal with some of these points while describing the operative procedures, which will, I hope, be useful to the trainee and practising vascular surgeon.

1991   P. R. F. Bell

To Anne for her patience.

Contents

Chapter 1

Preoperative assessments prior to distal surgery

Introduction

Before an operation is performed in a patient with distal arterial disease it is important to recognise the variables that will make the operation a success or failure. These could broadly be listed as: preoperative, intra-operative and postoperative. Among the important factors are: adequacy of inflow, the level at which the anastomosis is being performed, the graft being used and the skill of the surgeon. It is not in the remit of this book to consider factors such as the general condition of the patient or medical treatment in any detail, but to concentrate on those aspects which may influence the success or failure of the procedure from the technical point of view, and these are the aspects which will be covered in most detail.

SHOULD THE OPERATION BE DONE AT ALL?

Clearly, if at all possible every effort should be made to try and save the leg and this is nearly always the case when the obstruction lies in the proximal popliteal artery or even below the knee. However, if the disease is very distal with little or no run-off, then the question of whether or not to operate is important and needs to be answered objectively. A successful distal procedure in an old patient is a good operation and avoids amputation. However, a failed distal procedure merely exposes the patient to the psychological trauma of a second operation—usually an amputation, which is often at a higher level than would have otherwise been necessary.[1] Selection of patients for very distal procedures in particular becomes very important and every effort should be made to ensure that a successful operation is possible. If it is not going to be possible, then an amputation below the knee as the original procedure would be best for the patient. Of course, if there is any doubt about success then a reconstructive procedure should be performed.

Successful salvage has never been defined, but graft patency and limb preservation for at least one year would be acceptable, although some authors would expect less than this. At this point in time it is difficult to be sure which operations are and are not destined to fail. Clearly, if the patient's gangrene is extensive and includes the forefoot, the chances of a successful outcome are relatively poor. If, however, the process has not reached the forefoot and, in particular, if the patient's own long saphenous vein is available, then the chances of success are much better. There are, however, many patients in whom gangrene affects only the toes and where the chances of operative success are unknown. In these patients adverse factors would include the lack of a long saphenous vein, the presence of diabetes and the finding of a high peripheral resistance at operation.

PREOPERATIVE PREPARATION

Many of these patients are old and frail and careful attention to their general condition is essential. Many are having surgery to save the leg, so this procedure is essential and they must be made 'fit' for it. Heart failure must be treated, arrhythmias controlled and evidence of recent myocardial ischaemia elicited by ECG. The blood pressure should not be lowered too much as this can make rest pain worse, and certain drugs such as beta blockers should be stopped prior to surgery. Diabetes should, of course, be controlled and the chest cleared as far as possible by vigorous physiotherapy. It is not the remit of this book to describe medical treatment in any detail and collaboration with an interested physician and anaesthetist is very important and will reduce mortality. If the patient cannot tolerate a general anaesthetic, spinal or local anaesthesia is often applicable.

ANTIBIOTICS

The best combination of antibiotics to cover vascular procedures remains unknown. Because the consequences of infection are disastrous, however, some form of prophylaxis is necessary— exactly what this should be and how long it should last remains an open question. Because staphylococci are frequently implicated in such infections, some combination containing cloxacillin has been popular in the past. More recently, broad-spectrum antibiotics said to cover most organisms are being investigated. It is probably adequate to use one of the cephalosporins and give one injection with the premedication to cover most procedures. When infection or gangrene are present, a full course of treatment is probably needed, using a broad spectrum of agents which will usually include gentamicin, cloxacillin and metronidazole.

Possibly of more importance is preoperative preparation of the wound site because of the high incidence of *Staphyloccus epidermidis* infection in chronically infected grafts. The area to be incised should be painted with an alcohol containing antiseptic solution before the patient is taken to theatre. In addition, a bath containing an antiseptic prior to theatre is probably helpful. Antibiotics are, of course, particularly useful if artificial grafts are being used.[2]

VEIN MAPPING

There is no doubt that autologous vein gives the best results, particularly when grafts are placed to below knee vessels. For this reason, when deciding about the suitability of a patient for such procedures, the availability of a suitable vein is important. The long saphenous vein can be located either by venography using non-ionised contrast medium, or preferably by Duplex scanning.[3] Duplex is a better method as it is non-invasive and much more flexible, allowing the operator to mark exactly where the vein is on the skin. Knowing where the vein is allows a precise incision to be made over it and avoids undermining of skin flaps, which adds to morbidity by causing poor wound healing. In addition, if the saphenous vein is not present or inadequate, then suitable arm veins or the short saphenous vein can be marked out in a similar way. If a reversed saphenous vein is being used then it should probably be at least 4 mm at its smallest diameter. However, for in situ grafts a vein measuring 2 mm at its distal end can be used successfully.

IS THE INFLOW ADEQUATE?

Arteriography is the only investigation used by many surgeons to examine the aortoiliac segment. As a large number of patients have multisegment disease (Fig. 1.1), the importance of an adequate inflow prior to doing a distal operation is obvious. In any patient where there is clinical doubt about the femoral pulse or the appearance of the proximal segment on angiography, an inflow test should be performed. Unfortunately, there is no simple, non-invasive technique for assessing adequate inflow. Although a large number of publications have appeared purporting to show that Doppler waveform analysis using various measurements can separate patients who have significant aortoiliac disease from those who do not, sub-sequent investigations have not borne them out.[4] There have been various phases where pulsatility index, La Place transform analysis, and principal component analysis have been in vogue, but these tests are only useful if there is no downstream disease. The only test which has withstood the test of time is unfortunately invasive, but does provide information on poor inflow and has come to be known as the *papaverine test*.[5]

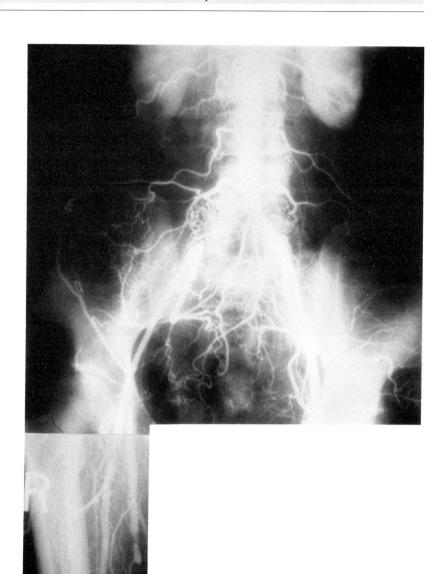

Fig. 1.1

An arteriogram of a patient with aortoiliac obstruction and occlusion of the superficial femoral artery on the right.

The papaverine test is based on the observation that a pressure difference across a stenosis is accentuated as flow is increased and is best done pre-operatively. A 21-gauge needle is inserted into the femoral artery on the affected side and attached to a strain gauge, which in turn is connected to a recording machine. For reference purposes, a second needle is inserted directly into a radial artery at the wrist and again attached to a second strain gauge which is connected to the same chart recorder, giving an estimate of the pressure proximal and distal to any potential stenosis of the aortoiliac segment. Alternatively, if the technology is available, then a catheter carrying two miniaturised pressure transducers can be inserted by the Seldinger route at arteriography (Fig. 1.2). This method is very useful provided that the catheter can be made to negotiate the stenosis in the iliac artery. If there is a resting pressure drop of more than 10 mmHg, this in itself is significant and no further test is necessary. However, if there is no resting difference, then 20 mg of papaverine is injected through the femoral artery needle and the tracing observed for the next 2–3 minutes until it returns to normal (Fig. 1.3). Any decrease in pressure of greater than 20% or, perhaps more significantly, a drop of more than 15 mmHg indicates a proximal stenosis of significant hae-modynamic potential.[5] For the test to be accurate, it is important that an increase in flow does actually occur. This can be assessed by placing a Doppler over the femoral artery and measuring an increase in velocity. It is not, however, usually necessary to do this in practice. If this test is positive, then the patient who is having the test because of a suspicious arteriogram or clinical findings needs to have a proximal procedure before/at the same time as/ instead of the distal graft being planned. Under these circumstances angioplasty is probably the method of choice.[6] Failure to improve the inflow could lead to failure of a distal operation.

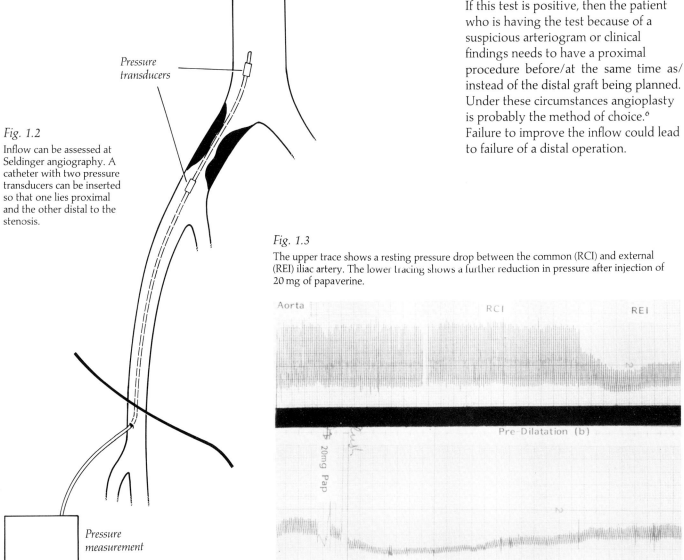

Pressure transducers

Fig. 1.2

Inflow can be assessed at Seldinger angiography. A catheter with two pressure transducers can be inserted so that one lies proximal and the other distal to the stenosis.

Pressure measurement

Fig. 1.3

The upper trace shows a resting pressure drop between the common (RCI) and external (REI) iliac artery. The lower tracing shows a further reduction in pressure after injection of 20 mg of papaverine.

Aorta   RCI   REI

20mg Pap

Pre-Dilatation (b)

Another non-invasive method of assessing inflow is to measure the 'rise time' of the femoral pulse. This method has been found useful in initial studies and necessitates the use of a transducer applied to the femoral artery.[7] It can be influenced by the state of the artery and its lack of elasticity, but could become useful in future if shown to be as accurate as direct pressure measurement.

LOCATING THE CORRECT ARTERY TO APPROACH FOR DISTAL PROCEDURES

Preoperative arteriography may not show any distal vessels in some patients with distal disease and rest pain. This does not mean there are none available, but knowing where to make the initial exploratory incision can be difficult. Two methods may be helpful. The first is to try and detect a Doppler signal over the three vessels at the ankle (anterior tibial, posterior tibial and peroneal) with the legs dependent. If this fails, a second technique called pressure generated run-off (PGR) can be used.[8] The principle of this test is to apply a sudden intermittent pressure to the vessels of the calf using a cuff and to

listen for the signal generated over each vessel at the ankle (Fig. 1.4). In this way, the vessel with the strongest signal can be explored as a potential site for the distal anastomosis. This method is explained in more detail in the chapter on femorocrural procedures. It may be possible to measure preoperative peripheral resistance using this test.

The importance of ensuring that the patient is as fit as possible, that the inflow is adequate and that the possibility of distal reconstruction is investigated by dependent Doppler or PGR cannot be overestimated. The margins for error, particularly for crural procedures, are so small that all of the factors which contribute to failure must be examined before proceeding.

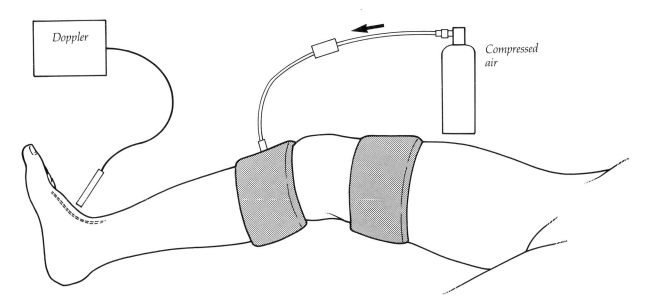

Fig. 1.4

Measuring pressure generated run-off. A cuff is intermittently inflated, generating a signal in the calf arteries which can be detected at the ankle by Doppler.

REFERENCES

1   Dardik H, Khan M, Dardik I, Susman B, Ibrahim I M 1982 Influence of
    failed bypass procedures on conversion of below knee to above knee
    amputation levels. Surgery 91: 64–69
2   Johnson J A, Coghill T H, Strutt P J, Grandersen A E 1988 Wound
    complications after infrainguinal bypass. Classification, predisposing
    factors and management. Archives of Surgery 123: 859–862
3   Bagi P, Schroder T, Selleson H, Lorentzen J E 1989 Real time B mode
    mapping of the greater saphenous vein. European Journal of Vascular
    Surgery 3: 103–107
4   Macpherson D S, Evans D H, Bell P R F 1984 Common femoral artery
    Doppler waveform: a comparison of three methods of objective
    analysis with direct pressure measurements. British Journal of Surgery
    71: 46–49
5   Quin R D, Evans D H, Bell P R F 1975 Haemodynamic assessment of
    the aortoiliac segment. Journal of Cardiovascular Surgery 16:
    586–589
6   Murie J A 1988 Percutaneous transluminal angioplasty and vascular
    surgery for lower limb ischaemia. British Journal of Surgery 75:
    1051–1053
7   Green L, Taylor A D, Greenhalgh R M 1987 Femoral artery rise time:
    an objective test for aortoiliac disease. European Journal of Vascular
    Surgery 1: 121–129
8   Beard J D, Scott D J A, Evans M, Skidmore R, Horrocks M 1988 Pulse
    generated run off: a new method of determining calf vessel patency.
    British Journal of Surgery 75: 361–363

Chapter 2

Intraoperative procedures

General principles

Results, as in every branch of surgery, will be best if undue trauma to tissues is avoided. At all times, therefore, the tissues should be dissected with scissors or scalpel and the temptation to use undue force should be resisted. Exposure should always be adequate, there is no place for keyhole surgery during vascular operations. It is usually wise to make sure that you have adequate control of the vessels you are operating on and this is achieved by encircling the vessel with a silastic sling, or if it is a small artery, with a tie. If this is done, then should a clamp inadvertently come off the vessel can easily be controlled by gentle traction on the appropriate sling. Vascular clamps should be used carefully when occluding a vessel, bearing in mind that many of the larger arteries are calcified and undue pressure with a clamp will lead to fracture of the vessel wall and damage which may not be retrievable. In the same way, undue pressure on a distal vessel can cause occlusion and lead to what was a reasonable run-off becoming an impossible situation. Smaller vessels, such as those in the lower limb below the knee, should not, if possible, be clamped—instead, gentle traction using the silastic sling is all that is required to arrest haemorrhage. In a situation where you are not sure about the potential damage to vessels from clamping, a good technique is to insert a Fogarty catheter (no. 3 size) with a three-way tap on one end: this will allow control over the bleeding by inflation of the balloon, without undue damage to the vessel.

HEPARINISATION

The use of heparin varies considerably in different centres. Some surgeons inject heparinised saline into the recipient and proximal artery as and when required. An alternative, which avoids the need for frequent injections of heparin, is to give the patient a sufficient dose intravenously to maintain generalised heparinisation. The advantage of this is that it obviates the need to inject heparinised saline into the vessel at intervals. The disadvantage, of course, is that the patient may bleed unduly during the operative procedure and after the clamps have been released. The reversal of heparin under these circumstances can lead to hypotension and can therefore be dangerous. Occasionally a patient may be sensitive to bovine heparin in particular and develop heparin-induced thrombosis due to platelet aggregation. My own preference is to use heparin given intravenously and not reverse it once the operation has been completed unless there is some overriding reason to do so. Either local or systemic heparinisation is acceptable and the choice will depend upon the particular prejudice of the operating surgeon. Most clinicians give an arbitrary dose of 5000 units systemically, which, from a practical point of view, is probably acceptable. However, studies have shown that measurements should be made intraoperatively to control activity accurately.[1]

MEASUREMENT OF RUN-OFF

Uniplanar arteriography is generally used to assess the adequacy of run-off, the presence of a vessel with continuity to the pedal arch being generally regarded as a good indicator of likely operative success. For popliteal reconstructions, the more run-off vessels there are, the better will be the long-term results. When dealing with distal anastomoses, however, the arteriogram alone is seldom sufficiently accurate to allow a judgement to be made and pre-reconstruction on-table arteriograms may show numerous areas of atheroma distal to the chosen reconstruction site, the significance of which remains uncertain. For these reasons, in *crural* anastomoses an objective assessment of the run-off by measuring peripheral resistance is important.

Three different techniques have been described for doing this, one of which is more a predictor of success or failure *after* reconstruction is complete.[2] The other two, however, could be used depending upon the availability of equipment. Our own technique utilises the patient's own blood and depends on measuring the peripheral resistance using arbitrary units of pressure.[3]

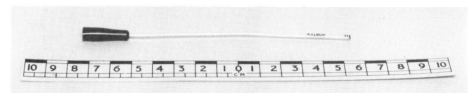

Fig. 2.1
Soft blunt silastic catheter inserted through a small arteriotomy into the artery chosen for the reconstruction.

Technique

Using preoperative arteriography or intra-arterial DSA, the chosen vessel is approached as described in the relevant section on distal procedures (p. 155). After exposure of the artery a soft cannula (Fig. 2.1) is inserted and blood withdrawn. The cannula allows blood to be pumped into the artery while the pressure in the system is measured. After insertion, which must be done carefully through a small arteriotomy without damaging the artery (Fig. 2.2), an on-table arteriogram is then performed through the catheter in order to confirm that the vessel is of reasonable calibre and, if possible, extends to the foot (Fig. 2.3). In that event, the catheter can then be connected to a pump (Fig. 2.4), which allows blood to be injected through the cannula at a fixed flow rate.

Fig. 2.3

A prereconstruction on-table arteriogram of the peroneal artery exposed after removal of a portion of the fibula.

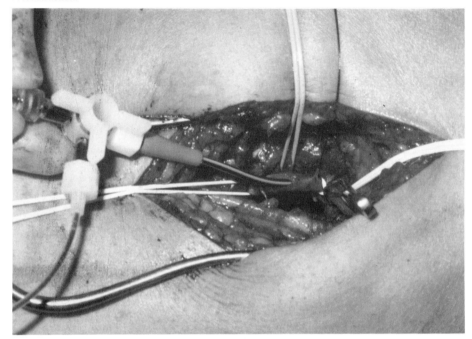

Fig. 2.2
The cannula is carefully inserted into the chosen artery without causing damage to it.

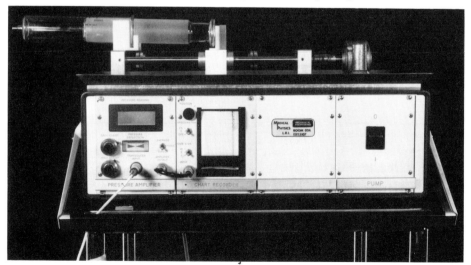

Fig. 2.4
The Harvard pump with the glass syringe on top used for injecting blood into the artery at a constant flow (100 ml/min).

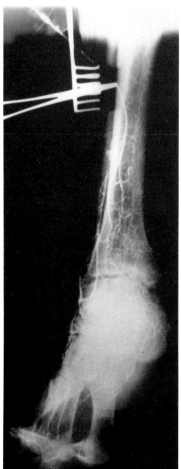

Once the vessel has been successfully entered, a needle is placed into the femoral vein in the groin for reference purposes (this is not essential) and 100 ml of blood is removed from the femoral artery using a heparinised glass syringe. The syringe is placed in the pump and the blood injected at a constant flow rate of 100 ml/min into the cannula which is in the recipient vessel (Fig. 2.5). Once a stable pressure is reached, papaverine (20 mg) is injected through a three-way tap into the pumped blood and the pressures again measured to assess the effect of vasodilatation. The peripheral resistance in arbitrary peripheral resistance units is measured using the formula:

$$\frac{\text{Peripheral}}{\text{resistance}} = \frac{\text{AV pressure difference}}{\text{Flow}}$$

(1 peripheral resistance unit PRU = 1000 mPRU)

Initial studies have shown that for femorodistal grafts, if the resistance is in excess of 1400 mPRU then the graft is unlikely to succeed.[3] The test is not very useful for femoropopliteal grafts.

It is important to recognise that this measurement is not too difficult to make, but does add time to the procedure. If it can be made, however, it gives an objective indication of outflow which, when taken with poor on-table arteriography and other adverse risk factors, such as gangrene, age, diabetes, etc., would suggest that an amputation should be performed as the definitive treatment in some cases. The test only gives an approximate idea of 'inoperable' cases and there is as yet no 'black and white' test available.

Another technique of measuring resistance is to use a spring-loaded syringe (Fig. 2.6) which is calibrated with a strain gauge to produce an infusion pressure of 100 mgHg. The

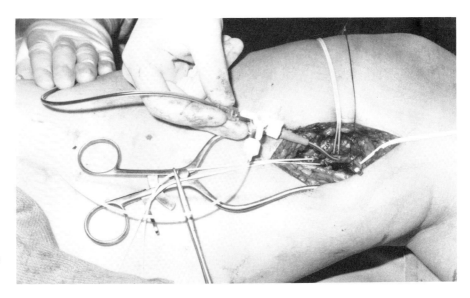

Fig. 2.5
Heparinised blood being pumped into the recipient vessel.

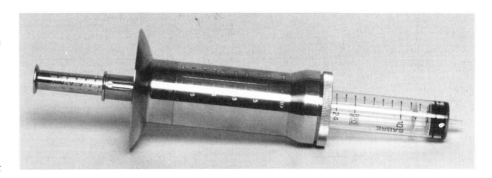

Fig. 2.6
Spring-loaded calibrated metal syringe which can be used to measure resistance.

time taken to inject 20 ml of blood into the recipient artery through a cannula at this pressure is then measured and the resistance read from calibrations on the barrel of the syringe. Using this technique, again a resistance between 1200 and 1500 mPRU is associated with poor long-term results.[4] This method may be simpler than using a pump, but it is less accurate.

ON-TABLE ARTERIOGRAPHY

Completion angiography is still the best method of assessing the result of the operation (Fig. 2.7) and, in cases where distal vessels have not been shown on preoperative angiography, an angiogram done prior to deciding the level of distal grafting is also important (Fig. 2.8) and improves results.[5] Post-operative arteriography is not done by some surgeons because they feel that it occupies too much time and exposes the person concerned to radiation hazards and is generally unnecessary. None of these statements is true.

Technique

If preoperative angiography has not shown a good distal vessel; the chosen artery should be exposed and controlled with silastic slings and a small butterfly needle inserted. It may be necessary to bend the barrel of the needle slightly before it can be placed into the artery easily and care should be taken to pass the needle slowly in order to avoid damage to the intima. If the wound is deep, the plastic wings of the needle can be approximated and grasped to effect easy entry, or they can be cut off. Once the needle has been placed in the artery, it should be attached to the skin with a

suture in order to prevent displacement later (Fig. 2.9). If the peripheral resistance is being measured, the arteriogram can be obtained by using the cannula already in place (see earlier). A long piece of plastic tubing is connected to the butterfly needle or cannula, the length being sufficient to allow the surgeon to stand behind the radiographer, who will be taking the film and wearing a protective apron. Saline is injected down the tubing into the artery and efforts made to make sure that back-bleeding is present. A standard full size X-ray plate is next wrapped in a sterile towel and placed under the limb, the

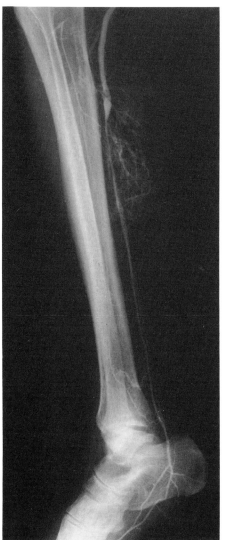

Fig. 2.7
Completion angiogram after PTFE grafting.

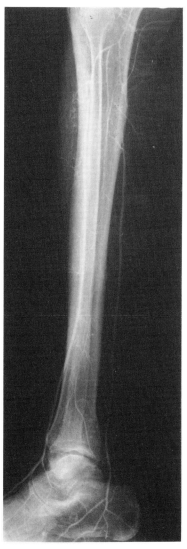

Fig. 2.8
No vessels were seen on preoperative angiography. On-table preoperative angiogram after injection into tibioperoneal trunk showing good distal crural vessels.

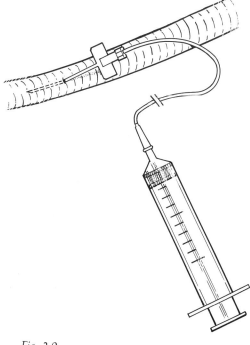

Fig. 2.9

position coinciding with the area of artery that needs to be seen (Fig. 2.10). Non-ionising contrast medium is next injected as rapidly as possible down the needle, and into the distal artery. When about 10 ml have been injected the injection continues and the film is taken while still injecting. The contrast is followed by an injection of saline and the film developed. If the X-ray has been performed to examine a graft following surgery, i.e. completion angiography, the principle is exactly the same except that the needle is inserted into the graft quite close to the distal anastomosis (Fig. 2.11). The graft is then clamped proximally prior to injecting contrast down it. If this is not done, then contrast will travel proximally and not outline the anastomosis. If this method is used, excellent on-table angiograms can be obtained (Fig. 2.12) and take approximately 5–10 minutes to achieve, provided the radiographer is sent for before the anastomosis is actually completed. The surgeon should remember to do this.

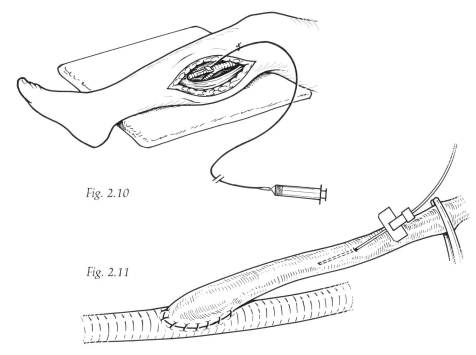

Fig. 2.10

Fig. 2.11

Fig. 2.12
Completion angiogram after in situ grafting.

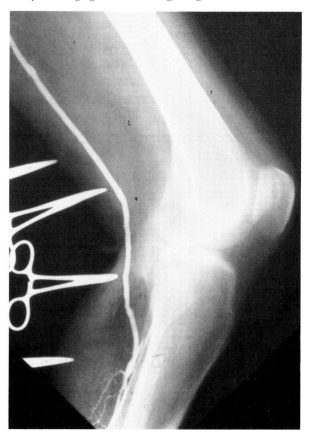

PASSAGE OF A FOGARTY CATHETER

Passing a Fogarty catheter is often an integral part of many vascular surgical procedures and may be necessary if completion angiography shows thrombus to be present distally. Various important points about its use need to be emphasised.

This simple exercise has revolutionised vascular surgery over the years and made it possible to remove thrombus from distal vessels at completion of, or prior to, an operation.[6] The catheter does, of course, come in a variety of sizes, and generally speaking nos 2 and 3 are most useful for the distal arteries in the leg. The catheter is removed from its sterile packaging and the internal wire, if present, removed. In these vessels the wire should not be left inside the catheter otherwise it will damage the artery. The catheter is attached to a 2 ml syringe and a trial inflation carried out without undue pressure. The balloon is then deflated and the catheter passed down the artery. This must be done carefully and gently. If the catheter comes to a halt, it must not be roughly pushed down the vessel as this will simply cause more damage. If it will not pass a narrow area there is no point in forcing it, and certainly no point in inserting the wire in order to get more 'push'. Once the catheter has gone down the artery as far as it can, the balloon should be gently inflated with the right hand, and the left hand used to remove the catheter (Fig. 2.13). This is done gradually, adjusting the pressure with the right hand so that the catheter can be removed relatively easily without causing severe pressure on the vessel. The same surgeon should inflate the balloon and remove the catheter. If clot is removed, the catheter must be passed again and passage must be continued until no further thrombus is removed and back-bleeding is obvious.

Problems that may occur

These usually relate to using too large a catheter in too small an artery, forcing the catheter through an area of obstruction or inflating the balloon too much: none of these should occur if the simple rules outlined above are followed. Very occasionally the balloon will not deflate; this can be tackled by measuring where the catheter is, after noting the marks on it, and either making a small incision over the area and deflating the balloon through the artery wall, or passing a wire down the inside of the catheter which will occasionally burst it. Generally speaking, overinflation in a small vessel is not to be recommended.

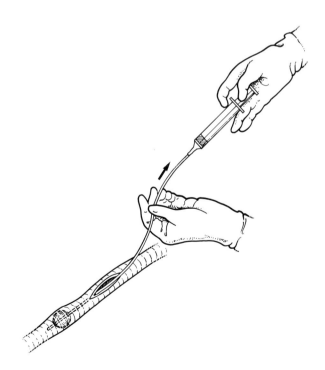

Fig. 2.13

GRAFTS AND SUTURES

Sutures

The availability of monofilament nylon sutures has made vascular anastomosis a much more satisfactory technical exercise. This, added to the variety of needles available, means that sutures should be available to the vascular surgeon to suit his individual needs. Monofilament nylon has the advantage of not causing an inflammatory reaction and is strong, but suffers from the disadvantage that it tends to retain the shape in which it is packed. This means that inadvertant knotting or snaring in instruments, etc. is or can be a problem. The recent availability of polytetrafluoroethylene (PTFE) suture is an advance in that this material has the advantages of monofilament nylon but remains flexible and does not necessarily conform to its packed shape. In addition, it is particularly useful when using PTFE grafts because it overcomes one of the problems of using that material, namely bleeding from needle holes. PTFE sutures tend to be elastic and bleed less when used with PTFE. In general, for anastomoses to the femoral or popliteal vessels, 5 or 6/0 sutures are most useful. For the distal profunda, crural or foot arteries, 6 or 7/0 sutures are best. These sutures will usually be attached to a variety of needles, which are taper cut, round bodied or cutting and come in a number of shapes and sizes. It is important that the operator acquaints himself with the various needles available in order to ensure that they suit his needs. In general, the needle should be taper cut, half circle and strong enough to allow passage through atheromatous vessels or tough graft materials.

Polytetrafluoroethylene (PTFE)

This material has now been available for a decade, but its initial promise has unfortunately not been sustained.[7] The original thick-walled variety has now been superseded by the introduction of

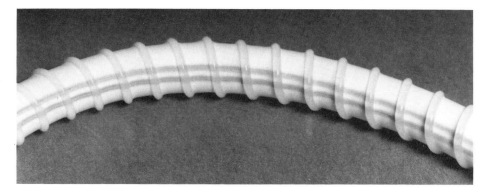

Fig. 2.14
Externally supported PTFE graft.

thin-walled PTFE grafts which are much easier to use. This material gives satisfactory results when used above the knee, but the results are worse when it is used below the knee. When it is anastomosed to the tibial vessels the results are relatively poor, but can be improved by the use of a vein patch at the distal anastomosis, which reduces intimal hyperplasia and improves results.[8] Recently, an external coiled support (Fig. 2.14) has been added to the grafts in order to prevent kinking when it crosses joints and this may improve results when using PTFE. It is important to remember that the material does not stretch and the arteriotomy has to be exactly the same size as the graft. If this is not the case then the graft will be narrowed and adequate flow prevented with consequent occlusion. Another problem is bleeding from suture holes at the anastomosis unless PTFE sutures are used. Bleeding can be stopped by applying haemostatic gauze with light pressure. For this reason, completion angiography should, if possible, be done through the native artery. Because the graft is non-wettable, another problem is that flow meters do not work, with perhaps the exception of the Doppler flowmeter.

Human umbilical vein

This graft is expensive but early results have shown it can be successful when used above or below the knee, but aneurysm formation is a potential hazard. It has been used in more distal situations and good results have been obtained by some authors.[9] Technically there are several problems which need to be emphasised. In particular, it is not possible to alter the position of the graft once the tunneller has been removed, so it has to be accurately placed. The thickness of the graft in relation to distal vessels can be a problem and there is no doubt that it is hard to use. When inserted subcutaneously, as it often is for below knee anastomoses, infection can occur due to erosion of the graft through the skin. It has a limited shelf life and is prone to aneurysm formation after several years of implantation.[10] Available comparative data suggest that it is superior to PTFE in femoropopliteal grafting, but this remains to be proved.[11]

Dacron

This graft is generally not successful when used as a femoropopliteal conduit, although there are some reports which suggest that it can be useful.[12] It can be effective, however, when used to join the iliac and popliteal arteries directly. As a general rule it is probably best not to use it for femoropopliteal or distal bypass procedures, but controlled trials comparing it with PTFE or human umbilical vein have not yet been done.

Bovine heterografts
These grafts have not been successful in the past because of aneurysm formation and thrombosis. However, a new graft made from calf artery is now undergoing trials and may prove to be more effective, although early results suggest that aneurysm formation may be a problem.[13]

These synthetic alternatives should therefore only be used where the long saphenous or other autologous vein is not available in the below-knee situation. If, however, a patient is being operated upon with an anastomosis above the knee, the question of using such material routinely should be addressed. As these patients are prone to further problems in future, it may be sensible to use artificial grafts rather than sacrifice the long saphenous vein which is much more useful if required for below-knee or coronary artery bypass grafting.

HAS THE OPERATION BEEN SUCCESSFUL?

Clearly it is important to decide as soon as possible if this is the case as otherwise reoperation due to graft occlusion will become necessary. A number of methods of assessing the operation are available, including on-table arteriography, measurement of flow before and after the injection of papaverine, measurement of foot volumetry using a pulse volume recorder, the use of Doppler to indicate forward flow, or measurement of peripheral resistance on completion of the anastomosis.

Arteriography
This technique has already been described earlier in this chapter.

Measurement of blood flow
An appropriate blood flow probe, either electromagnetic or the newer Doppler type, is placed around the graft and the flow measured. This can be a problem if PTFE is used because the material is an electromagnetic barrier and flow cannot be measured unless the probe can be placed around the artery above or below the insertion of a graft, which is often difficult. This is less of a problem with the Doppler flowmeter. After basal flow has been measured, papaverine is injected into the distal artery and any increase in flow assessed. Doubling of flow with papaverine suggests a good outcome and a basal flow of about 100 ml per minute should be achieved prior to the injection.

Pulse volume recorder
The foot is enclosed in an appropriate jacket to allow changes in volume to be measured. This is connected to a recorder, which provides information relating to pulsatile flow and gives an instant idea of revascularisation of the foot.[14] With the newer techniques it is rarely used now.

Doppler
Recently, the use of a sterile directional Doppler at operation placed on the graft gives an idea of reversed or forward flow. Adequate forward flow indicates that a satisfactory technical operation has been performed. The use of a Doppler flowmeter allied to the measurement of pressure in the graft will provide information on peripheral resistance, which relates to graft patency. Any graft with a high resistance can then be subjected to arteriography to find the cause.

Palpation of the pulses
If the leg is prepared correctly the ankle can be left exposed and palpation of the pulses after the operation is completed is a good indication that a satisfactory procedure has been performed, but this is not always possible, particularly with distal anastomoses. A sterile plastic bag placed over the foot also allows it to be seen and the colour assessed.

Drains
The insertion of a drain varies with surgeons. Some always insert one and others never do, saying they encourage infection. Data about their usefulness is not available, but I usually insert a fine suction drain at each infra-inguinal anastomosis and leave it for 24 hours.

REFERENCES

1   Porte R J, De Jong E, Knot E A R, de Maat M P M, Terpstra O T, Van
    Urk H, Groenland T H N 1987 Monitoring heparin and
    haemostasis during reconstruction of the abdominal aorta.
    European Journal of Vascular Surgery 1(6): 397–403
2   Ascer E, Veith F J, Morin L et al 1984 Quantitative assessment of
    outflow resistance in lower extremity arterial reconstructions.
    Journal of Surgical Research 37: 8–15
3   Parvin S D, Evans D H, Bell P R F 1985 Peripheral resistance
    measurement in the assessment of severe peripheral vascular
    disease. British Journal of Surgery 72: 751–753
4   Beard J D, Scott D J A, Evans J M, Skidmore R, Horrocks M 1988
    Blood flow measurement in clinical diagnosis. In: Price, Evans (eds)
    Conference Proceedings of the Biological Engineering Society,
    pp 64–68
5   Patel K R, Semel L, Claus R H 1988 Extended reconstruction rate for
    limb salvage with intraoperative pre reconstruction angiography.
    Journal of Vascular Surgery 7: 531–538
6   Rutherford R B, Jones D N, Bergentz S E et al 1988 Factors affecting
    the patency of infrainguinal bypass. Journal of Vascular Surgery 8:
    236–246
7   Quinones-Baldrich W J, Busuttil R W, Baker D et al 1988 Is the
    preferential use of polytetrafluoroethylene grafts for femoro-
    popliteal bypass justified? Journal of Vascular Surgery 8: 219–229
8   Miller J H, Foreman T K, Ferguson L, Faris I 1984 Interposition vein
    cuff for anastomosis of prosthesis to small artery. Australian and
    New Zealand Journal of Surgery 54: 283–286
9   Dardik H, Baker R E, Meinaghan M et al 1982 Morphological and
    biological assessment of longterm human umbilical vein implant
    used as a vascular conduit. Surgery, Gynecology and Obstetrics
    154: 17–26
10 Dardik H, Miller N, Dardik A et al 1988 A decade of experience with
    the gluteraldehyde-tanned human umbilical cord vein graft for
    revascularisation of the lower limb. Journal of Vascular Surgery 7:
    336–347
11 Eickhoff J H, Buchardt Hansen H J, Bromme A et al 1983 A
    randomised clinical trial of PTFE versus human umbilical vein for
    femoropopliteal bypass surgery: preliminary results. British Journal
    of Surgery 70: 85–89
12 Moseley J G, Marston A 1986 A 5-year follow up of Dacron
    femoropopliteal bypass grafts. British Journal of Surgery 73:
    24–28
13 Schroder H, Imig H, Peiper U, Neidel J, Petereit A 1988 Results of
    bovine collagen vascular prosthesis (Solcograft P) in infra-inguinal
    positions. European Journal of Vascular Surgery 2: 315–323
14 May A R L 1980 Monitoring femoropopliteal arterial reconstruction
    with the pulse volume recorder. In: Barr, Woodcock (eds)
    Diagnosis and monitoring in surgery. Wright, Bristol, pp. 149–153

Chapter 3

Postoperative care

Introduction

As already mentioned, these patients are ill and prone to early cardiac complications. They should be monitored in a high-dependency area or ITU for 24 hours after surgery and then watched carefully for several days until they stabilise. Antibiotics will not usually be continued unless there is a specific reason to do so, and a careful watch for cardiac or respiratory failure will be necessary. Early ambulation is to be encouraged and any drains that may have been inserted should be removed within 24 hours. For artificial grafts, antiplatelet agents or oral anticoagulants are sometimes used and there is some evidence that this is necessary for artificial grafts below the inguinal ligament.[1]

GRAFT OCCLUSION

If the graft occludes in the first few post-operative days, one attempt at un-blocking it is acceptable provided that there is thought to be a reasonable chance of success. If the outflow resistance at the original operation was very high (> 1400), unblocking it will probably not succeed and an amputation should be considered. If, however, the resistance was less than this and all other indications suggested success, then the graft should be explored and unblocked as soon as possible. To do this, the upper and lower anastomoses should be exposed and one side (usually the anterior wall) of the lower anastomosis opened. The patient should be heparinised and clot removed with a Fogarty catheter. Any technical problem should be carefully looked for and the anastomosis re-sutured. A completion angiogram should be done. Any specific lesion, such as a technical error, should be rectified. If necessary, a jump graft should be placed lower down the artery if there is a problem.

EARLY POSTOPERATIVE MONITORING

With distal grafts in particular it is often difficult to know if the graft has occluded as distal pulses are often absent. As a result, palpating the pulses is not enough and some objective form of graft assessment may give early warning of impending occlusion and allow successful reintervention. At present, apart from the use of externally applied Doppler probes, there is no easy way of doing this except perhaps by frequent postoperative Duplex assessment.

LATE MONITORING

In the first year, particularly if a vein graft has been used, patency should be assessed by Duplex or DSA in order to exclude a developing fibrous stenosis,[2] which can occur in up to 20% of cases and lead to premature graft occlusion (Fig. 3.1). Such lesions can, if discovered, easily be dealt with by angioplasty or surgery.[2] In addition, the importance of changing the various factors which caused the disease cannot be over-emphasised. The patient must stop smoking and should probably also lower their animal fat intake, particularly if the cholesterol level is raised. These parameters should be regularly monitored.

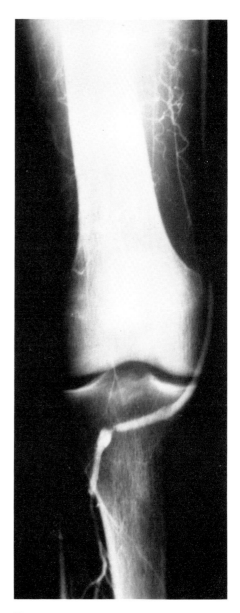

Fig. 3.1
Fibrous stricture in the lower third of an in situ vein graft three months postoperatively.

REFERENCES

1   Clyne C A C, Archer T J, Atuhair L K, Chant A D B, Webster J H H 1987 Random controlled trial of a short course of aspirin and dipyridamole (Persantin) for femorodistal grafts. British Journal of Surgery 74: 246–249
2   Grigg M J, Wolfe J H N, Tovar A, Nicolaides A N 1988 The reliability of Duplex derived haemodynamic measurements in the assessment of femorodistal grafts. European Journal of Vascular Surgery 2: 177–181

Chapter 4

General operative techniques used in various procedures

Introduction

As a rule the suture should always be passed from the inside of the artery to the outside, this avoids damage to the intima and prevents the separation of atheromatous material from the vessel wall. The artery should never be held firmly with forceps: a good technique is either to place the forceps inside the artery to provide counter traction without actually gripping the wall, or to hold the adventitia on the outside of the artery and provide counter traction in this way. It is important, particularly in small vessels, to evert the edges and thereby present the blood stream with a smooth uniform surface. For small anastomoses, magnifying loupes are very important and will minimise technical errors. If the vessels are small, interrupted sutures at the heel and toe will generally prevent a stenosis and give a better result. Never endarterectomise the vessel unless it is essential and do not try to stretch the graft to fit a large hole in the artery—reduce the size of the arteriotomy or make the graft bigger by cutting it obliquely. Always avoid tension and never finish anastomoses to small vessels at the corner. The various methods of constructing end-to-side and end-to-end anastomoses, which are the most commonly used in vascular surgery, will now be described.

END-TO-END ANASTOMOSIS

An end-to-end anastomosis is frequently required for the insertion of a bifurcated graft to the iliac arteries and in other reconstructions. If the vessel is large enough, a continuous stitch is all that is required. However, this is not the case for small vessels, such as those found near the ankle. The graft or vessel is cut across cleanly and double-ended sutures (the size of which will depend upon the size of the vessel) are inserted as shown in Figure 4.1. It is important to pass the needle from the inside to the outside of the artery thereby avoiding detaching atheromatous material. Both sutures are tied (Fig. 4.2) and one of them run along the front of the anastomosis taking small bites and using an everting technique. Once the anterior wall has been completed (Fig. 4.3) the stitch is tied to one of the other two sutures, thus completing the anterior wall of the anastomosis. Providing there is sufficient length, and there should usually be, the suture on the left (C) is then passed behind the vessel and the one on the right (D) taken towards the left, thereby turning the artery over and

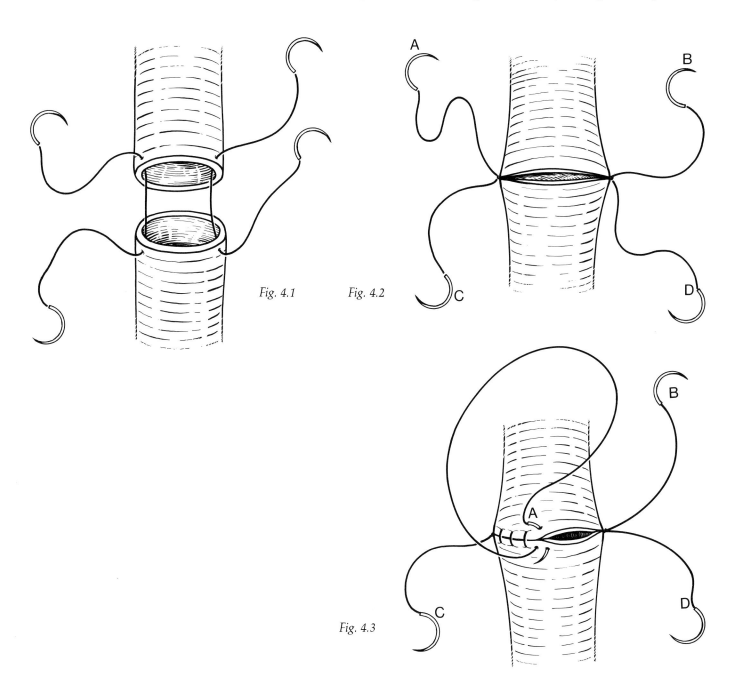

Fig. 4.1   Fig. 4.2

Fig. 4.3

exposing the posterior wall. The anastomosis is then completed by stitching from each end to the middle (Fig. 4.4) again using an everting technique. Once the middle is reached by both needles, the remaining sutures are tied to each other. If the vessels are small, such as those found at the ankle, and an end-to-end suture is being performed, then it is wisest to use an interrupted technique. Both vessels are first sewn together, as already described, with double-ended sutures, which are held with small bulldog clamps to provide a little tension. Interrupted sutures are then passed and tied sequentially, each one being held with a small bulldog clamp. As the process continues the vessel is turned over and the back wall completed (Figs 4.5, 4.6).

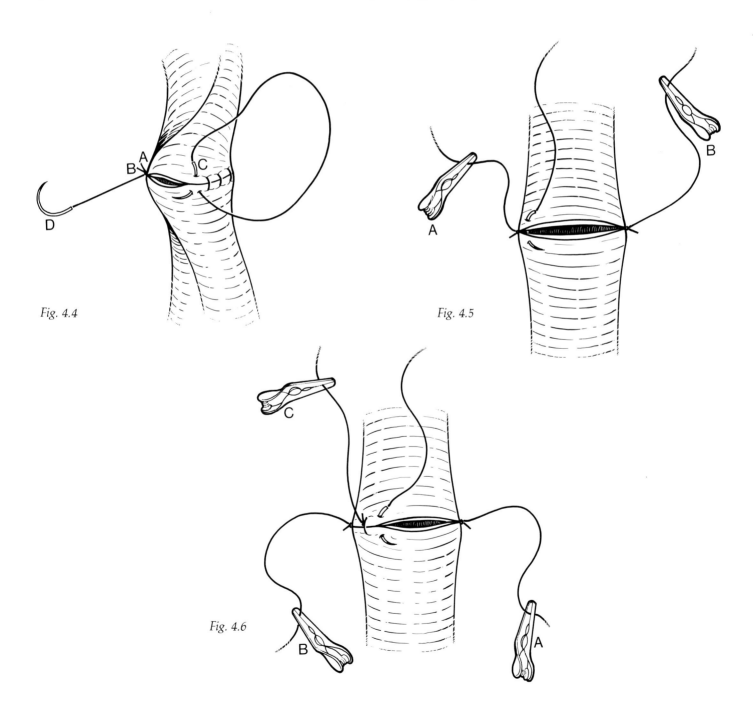

Fig. 4.4

Fig. 4.5

Fig. 4.6

Where the vessel cannot be turned, a different technique is necessary. In this situation it is best to pass a double-ended suture between the two ends at the back as shown in Figure 4.7. Again it is important to pass the needle from inside to the outside of the vessel. One of the needles is passed to the opposite side behind the vessel and the other is then used to stitch the back wall (Fig. 4.8). The needle is then passed from the outside to the inside and inside to outside in a succession of passes until the corner is reached (Fig. 4.9). Tension is then maintained on this needle and the process repeated for the opposite side of the back wall using the other needle. Once the side walls have been reached the stitch is continued around the front of each side of the artery and the sutures are then tied to each other. In this way it is not necessary to rotate the vessel.

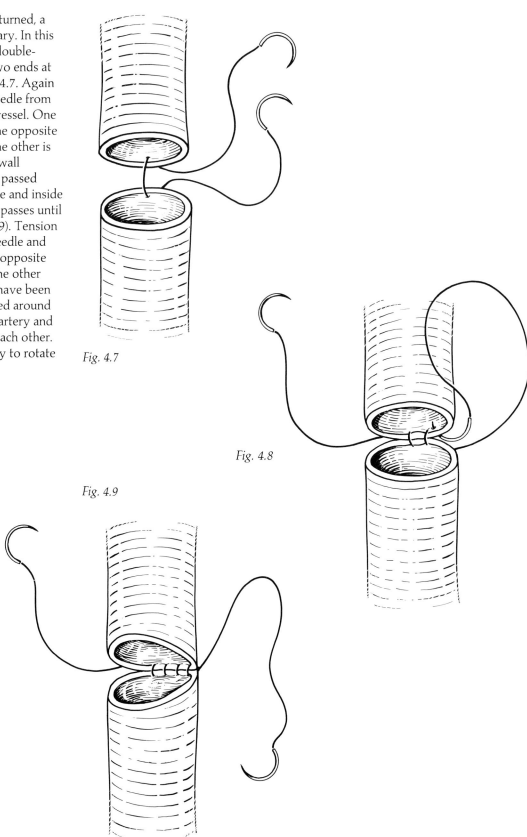

Fig. 4.7

Fig. 4.8

Fig. 4.9

END-TO-SIDE ANASTOMOSIS

These are probably the most common anastomoses used in vascular surgery and have the advantage that they do not disturb the recipient vessel unduly and allow a larger anastomosis to be made. The graft is first of all tailored by cutting it obliquely to fit the arteriotomy. The suture is then inserted from the inside to the outside of the vessel (Fig. 4.10) and the heel of the graft tied down to the recipient artery. One of the needles is then passed behind the graft, between it and the recipient artery, and the other used to sew one side of the anastomosis (Fig. 4.11). Again a continuous everting stitch is usually used and taken around the toe of the graft if the anastomosis is a large one, as is the case in most femoropopliteal or proximal procedures. Once the toe has been passed (Fig. 4.12), the rest of the anastomosis is completed with the other needle until it reaches the first needle to which it is tied. It is important to do the easiest side first as the second more difficult one then becomes simpler. Doing it the other way round makes for unnecessary difficulties.

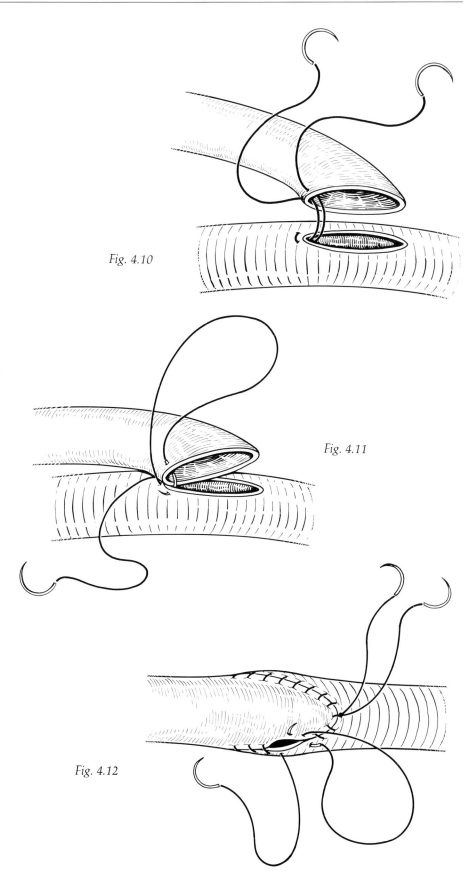

Fig. 4.10

Fig. 4.11

Fig. 4.12

An alternative technique is shown in Figure 4.13. In this situation, both the toe and the heel of the graft are stitched to the artery using double-ended sutures tied on the outside. Once this has been done the graft is stitched in place along one side and then the other, finishing in the middle of the anastomosis to avoid undue narrowing. This technique is probably the less versatile of the two and generally speaking it is better simply to stitch down the heel and work forward. If two sutures are used then flexibility is lost, although this is the best way to do the operation when learning the technique. Some authors favour a technique called parachuting, especially when large vessels are being sutured. This entails placing a number of sutures without pulling them tight until three or four have been inserted. They are then pulled tight collectively (Fig. 4.14). This method has the advantage that it allows accurate placing of the stitch, but can cause damage to delicate arterial walls when pulled too tightly. I do not personally use this method for this reason.

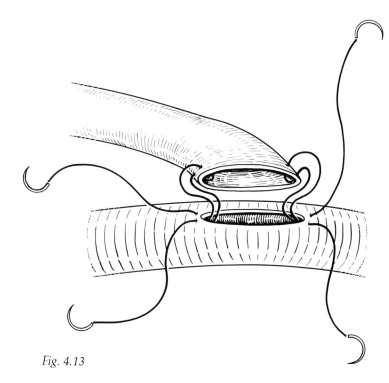

Fig. 4.13

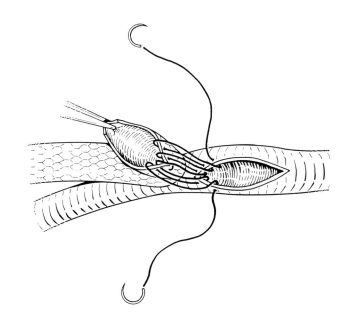

Fig. 4.14

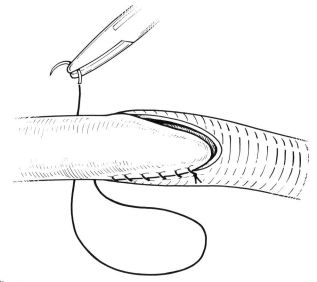

Fig. 4.15

If the end-to-side anastomosis has been constructed with small vessels, such as those at the ankle, then it is best to proceed as in Figures 4.15 and 4.16. Once again, a double-ended suture is inserted into the heel of the graft as previously shown and each suture taken down the sides (Fig. 4.15). The toe of the anastomosis is best completed, however, using a succession of interrupted sutures, which are tied only after they have all been inserted (Fig. 4.16). For small vessels, a useful tip is not to cut the graft to a point, as described later, but to take one corner of the graft, as in Figure 4.17, down to the apex of the arteriotomy and then tailor the other corner to suit the needs of the situation.

Fig. 4.16

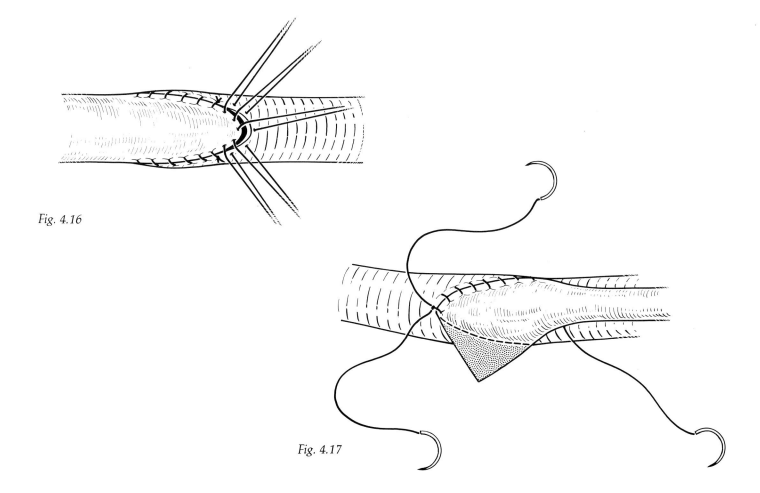

Fig. 4.17

Where there is disparity between the two ends of the graft, several different possibilities can be entertained. Firstly, as in Figure 4.18, the graft can be invaginated into the recipient artery as the suturing proceeds, and this is perfectly acceptable. Secondly (Fig. 4.19), the suture is arranged in such a way that narrower bites of artery in terms of width are taken of the small vessel and slightly larger ones of the bigger vessel and in this way the mismatch can be distributed evenly around the circumference. The last possibility is to cut the smaller of the two arteries obliquely and sew this oblique, and therefore larger hole, to the recipient vessel (Fig. 4.20).

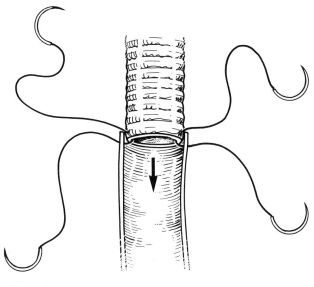

Fig. 4.18

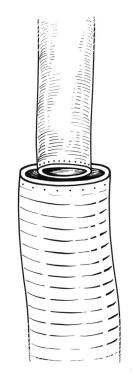

Fig. 4.19

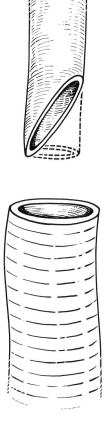

Fig. 4.20

ENDARTERECTOMY

Endarterectomy, apart from that practised for the carotid vessels, is generally not undertaken in other areas, although it is making a comeback in the aortoiliac segment.[1] It may be necessary to do a limited endarterectomy as part of an anastomosis. The affected area of the vessel is isolated by appropriate dissection and a longitudinal arteriotomy made (Fig. 4.21). Once the narrowed area has been crossed the incision in the artery is extended upwards and downwards until an area where the relatively normal vessel is encountered. Using a blunt ended instrument such as a Watson Cheyne dissector, the atheromatous material is separated from the muscular wall of the artery (Fig. 4.22). A plane can usually be found by dissection and the atheromatous plaque separated from the wall in a circumferential fashion. Once the thickened intima has been completely freed from the artery, it is divided proximally and distally (Figs 4.23 and 4.24) leaving behind an area of endarterectomised vessel.

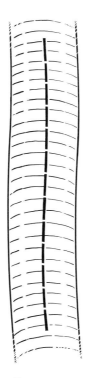

Fig. 4.21

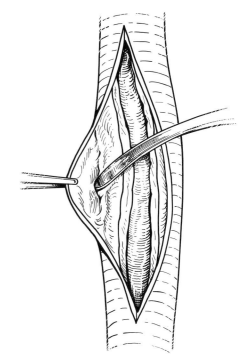

Fig. 4.22

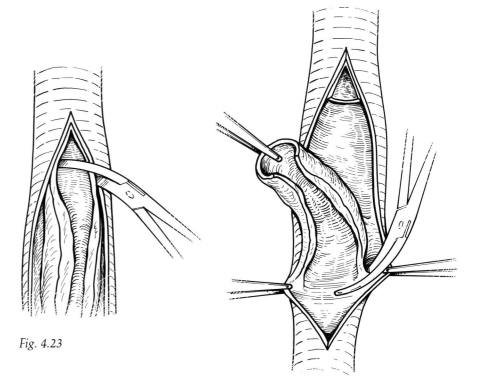

Fig. 4.23

Fig. 4.24

The proximal intima requires no attention; the distal layer does, however, sometimes need to be stitched down with circumferential sutures placed across the edge (Fig. 4.25). Double-ended sutures passed from the inside to the outside of the vessel are best for this purpose (usually 6 or 7/0). Once the endarterectomy has been completed, the defect is closed with a patch of vein or Dacron using continuous sutures to complete it (Fig. 4.26). It is important to ensure that the patch passes across the endarterectomised section and beyond where the intima becomes relatively normal again. In this way the step, particularly distally, so formed is not so serious an obstruction to the flow of blood and minimises thrombosis.

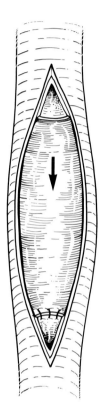

Fig. 4.25

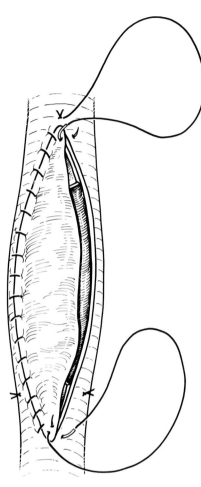

Fig. 4.26

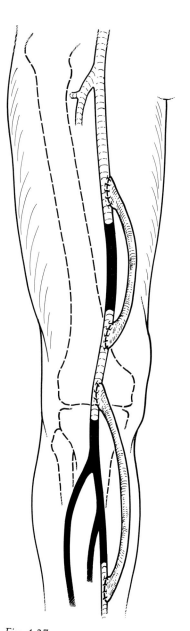

Fig. 4.27

SEGMENTAL GRAFTS

There is some evidence that long grafts of saphenous vein or artificial materials do not do as well as short segments of vessel, although a controlled trial to prove this point is not available.[2] It is therefore possible that areas of occlusion should be bridged by pieces of vein graft to give better long-term results (Fig. 4.27). This approach has the advantage that small pieces of vein can be used, such as those taken from the arm when saphenous vein might not be available. For this procedure, smaller areas of exposure are necessary and multiple incisions will be required. End-to-side anastomoses are usually done, disturbing the tissue and the vessels as little as possible, thereby maintaining collaterals.[3] Figure 4.27 is a diagram of a patient with multiple occlusions showing a segmental graft circumventing a femoral artery occlusion above the knee and a second one taken from this segment of popliteal artery to the anterior tibial lower down. This technique allows the placement of grafts isotopically and, although a large number of anastomoses are required, the eventual result may be superior.

SPECIAL TECHNIQUES USED FOR ARTERIAL TRAUMA

Trauma to arteries frequently accompanies fractures and leads to distal ischaemia. When recognised, this must be dealt with expeditiously, otherwise irreparable damage and ischaemia will occur to the leg.[4] The injury can take several forms, from complete rupture of the artery, contusion and thrombus formation or intimal fracture leading to secondary thrombosis and occlusion (Fig. 4.28). Remedial action will depend upon which injury is seen. Quite frequently a segment of vessel is destroyed completely and the ends retracted. If possible, when the artery is divided a primary end-to-end anastomosis should be performed, but only after appropriate excision of the damaged ends. This can sometimes be achieved by ligating one or two tributaries, but this should be kept to a minimum and if extensive ligation seems necessary, or if there is any sign of tension, a vein graft should be interposed between the two vessels. Whether a vein graft has been inserted or an end-to-end anastomosis performed, the technique is as described under the various methods of doing anastomoses on page 27. It is usually possible to rotate the graft or the vessel to do the appropriate procedure (Figs 4.29 and 4.30). If occlusion is due to an area of intimal destruction and stripping, then it may be possible to rectify matters without excising the artery. In this event a longitudinal arteriotomy is made across the contused area, after appropriately mobilising and controlling the artery. Loose atheroma is excised cleanly and the distal intima sutured down to the arterial wall (Figs 4.31 and 4.32), double-ended sutures are usually passed from the inside of the artery to the outside and placed individually in a circumferential fashion until the distal intima has been secured. When this has been done, the longitudinal arteriotomy is closed with a vein patch using continuous sutures (Fig. 4.33). It is vital that the patch passes across the shoulder where the intima has been stitched down. In general, it is best to excise the damaged artery (Fig. 4.34) and place a vein graft (Fig. 4.35).

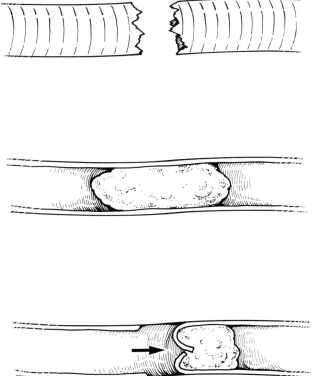

Fig. 4.28

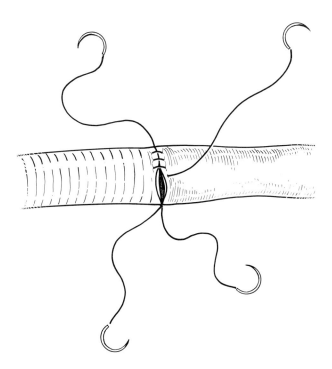

Fig. 4.29

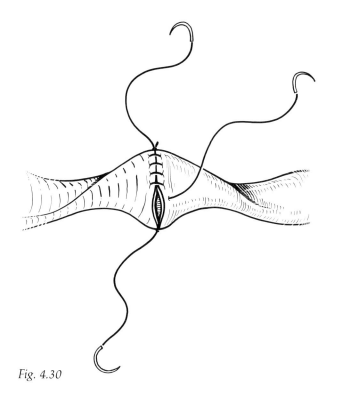

Fig. 4.30

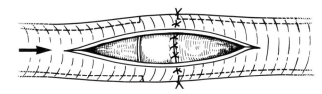

Fig. 4.31

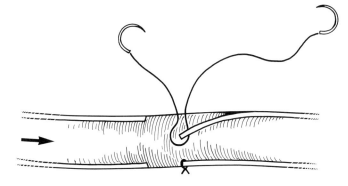

Fig. 4.32

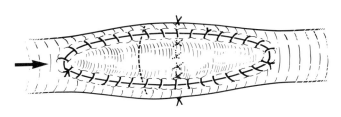

Fig. 4.33

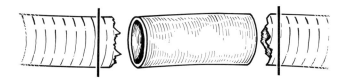

Fig. 4.34

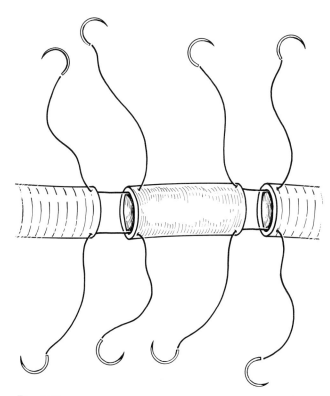

Fig. 4.35

INTRAOPERATIVE ANGIOPLASTY

This technique is not used by many surgeons, partly because they have not been trained to do it and partly because the screening equipment needed to use it properly is not always available in the operating theatre. In future it will undoubtedly be used more often, either alone[5] or with laser assistance in the operating theatre.[6] One can argue about the pros and cons of using this technique intraoperatively or prior to surgery; however, using it at surgery does have some advantages which include the removal of debris through the arteriotomy, thus avoiding distal embolisation, and the ability to put right any complications that might occur at the time. In spite of this argument, proximal lesions are probably best dealt with in the angiography suite where the equipment to do these techniques is available. The same arguments probably apply to short segments in the femoral artery, but possibly not to lesions over 10 cm in length. The main area of interest for intraoperative angioplasty, as yet largely unexplored, is probably the crural vessels, using balloons made for crural arteries. The arrival of the linear extrusion catheter[7] may make intraoperative angioplasty simpler and obviate the need for advanced screening equipment in the operating theatre. Conventional angioplasty techniques require the passage of a guide wire over which a suitably sized dilating balloon is passed. The linear extrusion method seeks to place the tip of the catheter at the origin of the stenosed segment. By appropriate pressure the extrusion balloon is slowly, as the name implies, forced into the narrow segment until it negotiates it completely, thereafter the balloon can be inflated to produce an angioplasty. The size of the balloon needed is first of all assessed by passing a latex sizing catheter up to the narrowed segment and measuring the volume of fluid needed to inflate the balloon to a size where it will just engage the adjacent 'normal' artery. This method needs extensive trial before its effectiveness can be assessed, but may be useful in those common stenoses seen in crural arteries.[8]

EMBOLECTOMY

This technique is often part of many vascular reconstructions where thrombus is thought to be present in the vessels distal or proximal to the anastomosis. It is also often used alone to remove thrombus causing acute ischaemia of the limb, the thrombus usually arising in the heart from the atrium, or a ventricular mural thrombus following myocardial infarction. The embolus is usually lodged below the inguinal ligament in the femoral or popliteal artery and fragments often also pass into the profunda femoris. Most of these patients are ill and a local infiltration anaesthetic is all that is needed but an anaesthetist should be available in case further procedures are necessary.

Procedure

The femoral vessels are first of all exposed, as described later in Chapter 10. The incision can be either oblique or vertical, but need not be as large as that required for a femoropopliteal graft. Much less of the vessel needs to be exposed than for a grafting procedure, but sufficient of the artery must be seen to allow control of the common femoral, superficial femoral and profunda femoris vessels. It is usually sufficient to expose the common femoral artery immediately above its bifurcation, the superficial femoral distal to this point and the origin of the profunda femoris. It is particularly important to expose the latter vessel as this needs to be thoroughly emptied of any thrombus. Silastic slings should be passed, as already described, for control of the vessel in intraoperative grafting, allowing enough space to apply a vascular clamp, particularly on the proximal common femoral artery. The patient will usually have been heparinised. If not, 5000 units of heparin are given systemically by the intravenous route. If the surgeon is reasonably sure that the cause of the ischaemia is an embolus, the vessel is clamped proximally and a small transverse incision made in the front of the common femoral artery opposite the point where the profunda femoris arises. This arteriotomy can be made with a scalpel or scissors and should just be large enough to allow thrombus to be removed, but not be so large as to almost transect the vessel. A transverse incision has the advantage that it can be closed easily without causing a stenosis. If there is any doubt about the possibility of an embolus and a possible graft being required later, then a vertical incision should be made in the same place slightly above the origin of the profunda femoris. This allows more flexibility for any further procedure that might be necessary, but it must be closed very carefully with a patch of vein or Dacron to avoid stenosis. A proximal vascular clamp will of course have been placed before the arteriotomy is made. If the diagnosis is correct, thrombus will usually be seen in the artery and a no. 3 Fogarty catheter selected and the central wire removed. The balloon is then inflated with saline from a 2 ml syringe to make sure it is intact. The balloon is then deflated and the catheter passed as in Figure 4.36. The catheter is passed first of all down the superficial femoral artery until it will pass no further. On no account should force be used for this manoeuvre. When it comes to rest, the level should be noted by the markings on the Fogarty catheter and the balloon expanded with saline using the right hand. The left hand is now used to grasp the catheter and withdraw it gently. The amount of distension of the balloon is controlled with the right hand in such a way that the removal of the catheter is smooth and done without undue pressure of force (Fig. 4.36). Thrombus will usually emerge with the catheter and the process *must* be repeated until no more thrombus is obtained and there is good back bleeding. The superficial femoral artery is then clamped or occluded by

tension on the sling and the process repeated with the profunda femoris artery. The catheter will not, of course, pass as far down this vessel. but it must be passed until all thrombus is removed and there is back bleeding. Once this has been done it must be ascertained that there is adequate inflow and this can be confirmed by releasing the proximal clamp. If there is any doubt the catheter, usually a larger one—no. 4 or 5—should be passed proximally. The arteriotomy is then closed with continuous or interrupted 5/0 Prolene if it is transverse, or, if there is any doubt about narrowing in the case of a vertical incision, a patch of vein or Dacron should be used to close it. Once the circulation has been restored, a completion angiogram is performed (see p. 15) by inserting a needle into the superficial femoral artery. If any thrombus remains, the vessel should be reopened and the process repeated until all thrombus has been removed and completion angiography found to be satisfactory. Alternatively, an arteriogram can be performed with one of the newer Fogarty catheters which has a second channel and, following adequate removal of thrombus, contrast can be injected down the second channel and a film obtained allowing subsequent closure of the vessel and completion of the procedure.

Problems with embolectomy
If good back bleeding or adequate clearance on completion angiography is not obtained, the wound must on no account be closed in the erroneous hope that all will be well. Angiography will have shown the presence or otherwise of a distal vessel and the popliteal artery below the knee should next be explored as described in Chapter 11. The main vessel above the trifurcation should be dissected and controlled with slings and a Fogarty catheter passed proximally. This will often result in thrombus, which may have been adherent, being removed. It should of course also be passed distally into as many of the crural branches as proves possible. If this also fails, then the patient will require a further procedure, which may be some form of grafting to the popliteal or crural vessels (Chs 11, 12 or 13). If this is not done then the patient may lose the limb.

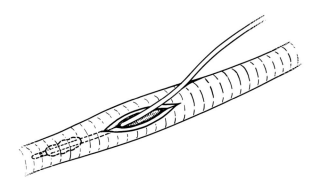

Fig. 4.36

REFERENCES

1   Willekens F G J, Wever J, Nevelsteen A et al 1987 Extensive
    disobliteration of the aorto iliac and common femoral arteries using
    the Le Veen plaque cracker. European Journal of Vascular Surgery
    1(6): 391–397
2   Ascer F, Veith F J, Gupta S K et al 1988 Short vein grafts: a superior
    option for arterial reconstructions to poor or compromised outflow
    tracts? Journal of Vascular Surgery 7(2): 370–377.
3   Largiader J, Peter M 1987 A surgical strategy for femoro-crural
    reconstruction. European Journal of Vascular Surgery 1(3): 205–213
4   Allen M J, Nash J R, Ionnides T, Bell P R F 1984 Major vascular injuries
    associated with orthopaedic injuries of the lower limb. Annals of the
    Royal College of Surgeons 66: 101–104
5   Pfeiffer R B, String S T 1986 Adjunctive use of the balloon dilatation
    catheter during vascular reconstructive procedures. Journal of
    Vascular Surgery 3: 841–845
6   Diethrich E B, Trimbadia E, Bahadir I 1989 Applications and limitations
    of laser assisted angioplasty. European Journal of Vascular Surgery
    3(1): 61–71
7   Fogarty T J, Chin A, Shoor P M, Blair G L, Zimmerman J J 1981
    Adjunctive intraoperative arterial dilatation: simplified instrumen-
    tation technique. Archives of Surgery 116: 1391–1396
8   Fogarty T J, Chin A K, Finn C J 1989 Peroperative luminal angioplasty.
    In: Greenhalgh R M (ed) Vascular surgical techniques. W B Saunders,
    London pp 319–326

Chapter 5

Profundaplasty

Introduction

This operation was first described by Natali[1] and popularised by Martin,[2] but since then its popularity has waned considerably and the indications for its use have become more specific. The profunda femoris artery is, of course, a vessel on which limb viability depends because it is frequently patent after occlusion of the superficial femoral. Whether or not its patency is sufficient to maintain the limb depends on a number of factors, such as adequate collaterals between it and the lower limb vessels and also the extent of distal disease. When the operation was first suggested, and also to a lesser extent since that time, the surgical procedure of profundaplasty using a wide patch over a distance of at least 2–3 cm, was thought to be capable of increasing limb blood flow irrespective of considerations such as those mentioned above. Because of its indiscriminate use, which did not produce improved limb salvage rates, the operation is now only done occasionally in some centres. However, profunda stenosis should be looked for routinely on arteriography, particularly using oblique views, otherwise a stenosis cannot clearly be seen (Fig. 5.1).

In a case where profundaplasty is indicated, it should be used as the results can be good, particularly in an old patient where a relatively minor procedure may save the leg. Generally speaking this is a patient who has minimal aortoiliac disease and distal disease of a type which precludes direct vascular intervention, but in whom a profunda stenosis is also present. Such a patient should be considered for the operation, particularly if objective evidence of significant obstruction is available. Angioplasty has not been extensively used in these patients, perhaps because of the technical difficulty of introducing a balloon so close to the bifurcation of the common femoral artery, although this problem can partly be avoided by approaching the lesion from the other side.

INDICATIONS FOR PROFUNDAPLASTY

The indications for this procedure have contracted since the initial description of the operation. In general, the patient will be elderly and there will be no inflow problem either on arteriography or on inflow testing. In addition, there will usually be evidence of distal disease with a poor run off and a definite stenosis of the profunda femoris artery (Fig. 5.1). In this situation, it usually means that the femoral artery has been occluded for some time and collateral flow has kept the leg intact. Increasing stenosis of the profunda orifice will have led to a deterioration in the condition of the foot so that rest pain or imminent gangrene is obvious. The operation is not usually worth considering in other situations and certainly not for claudication. A short profundaplasty is often, however, part of an aorto-bifemoral grafting procedure. The lower anastomosis of such grafts should be placed across the origin of the profunda femoris artery so that proper exposure of this vessel, as described later, will be required. Occasionally the upper end of a distal graft will be taken from the same area, particularly if there is some profunda stenosis present.

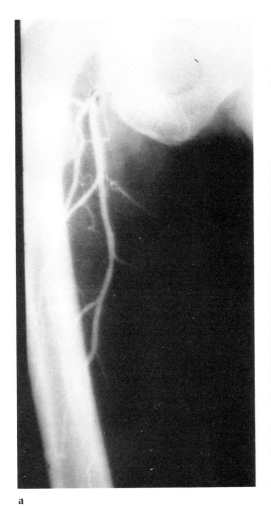
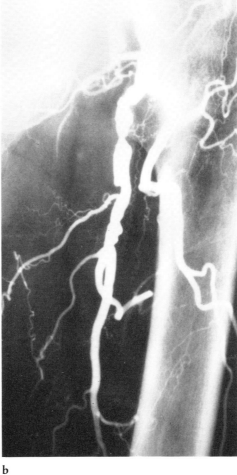

a

b

Fig. 5.1
A single significant stenosis of the origin of the profunda femoris artery can be seen in *A*. In *B* there are multiple stenoses of the profunda femoris which may or may not be significant.

THE OPERATION

The patient will usually be lying on the back. The lower half of the abdomen and the leg down to the ankle should be prepared and cleaned with an appropriate antiseptic solution so that when the towels are applied the entire limb is available and in the operative field. The foot can generally be covered, either with a towel, an orthopaedic sock, or a sterile transparent plastic bag. The reason for exposing the abdomen above the inguinal ligament and the limb distally is in case access is required to proximal or distal vessels. The incision is either oblique or vertically placed over the femoral artery extending across the inguinal ligament proximally and distally for 8–10 cm (Fig. 5.2). The length can be varied depending upon the access required. Once the incision has been deepened through the skin, the fascia over the femoral pulse is incised using a pair of toothed forceps and curved dissecting scissors. A self-retaining mastoid type retractor can be inserted and is useful for this part of the operation (Fig. 5.3). Care must be taken not to damage the long saphenous vein on the medial side. Any filamentous tissue resembling lymphatics should be ligated with fine absorbable ligatures (3/0), otherwise the operation should proceed by using sharp dissection. If the pulse is not palpable, the femoral vessels can usually be felt as longitudinal structures which can be rolled by the finger. The artery is approached by picking up the fascia and fat over it and incising it longitudinally. The medially placed femoral vein is not usually disturbed and the laterally placed femoral nerve is not seen. The correct layer is finally reached, at which point the artery wall is clearly seen as a slightly shiny circular structure (Fig. 5.4). The superficial circumflex vessels may sometimes be seen passing across the femoral artery and vein and need division and ligation.

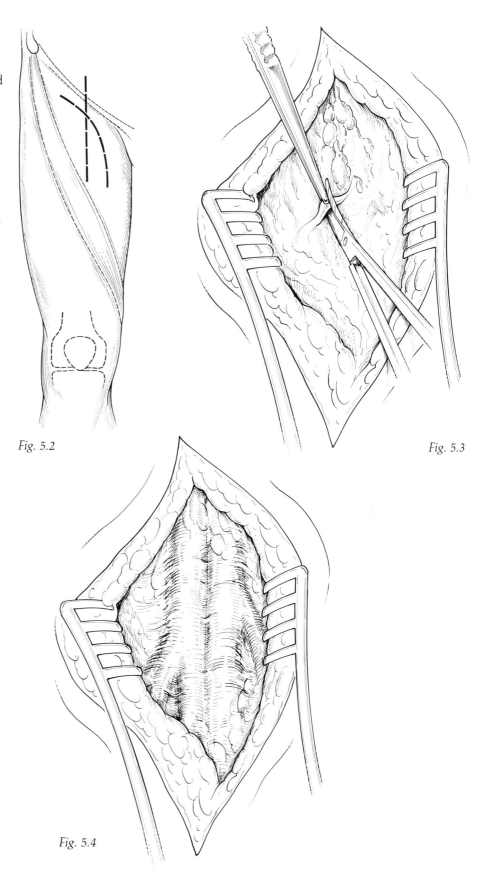

Fig. 5.2

Fig. 5.3

Fig. 5.4

By grasping the fascia immediately
overlying the artery with a pair
of forceps, it is possible to dissect
on each side of the vessel using
blunt curved scissors over a short area
of 1–2 cm (Fig. 5.5). Once this has been
achieved, an appropriately curved clamp
is passed around the artery (Fig. 5.6) and
a silastic sling drawn around it (Fig. 5.7).
Depending on the level of the bifurcation, either the superficial femoral
or common femoral artery will be the
first vessel to be encountered. Once the
sling has been placed around the artery,
gentle traction on it will allow the dissection to proceed distally and
proximally using scissors as before. By
gently opening and closing the scissors,
any branches will be discovered before
they are cut. There are often one or two
small branches passing laterally from the
common femoral artery, but none
usually from the first few centimetres of
the superficial femoral artery. The
junction between common and
superficial femoral artery can easily be
seen because the vessel narrows significantly as it becomes the superficial
femoral. This point is the clue to the
origin of the profunda femoris artery. By
dissecting the fascia around the
narrower superficial femoral artery in
the same way as described for the
common femoral, a lahey or curved
forcep is used to pass a sling around the
origin of this vessel (Fig. 5.8). By gentle
traction on both sets of slings, it is then
possible to see the origin of the profunda femoris artery. This vessel usually
passes laterally, occasionally medially
and sometimes directly behind the
superficial femoral artery. Using sharp
dissection the origin of the profunda
femoris is then encircled carefully, again
using a curved forcep such as a lahey
forcep (Fig. 5.9). Gentle traction on this
sling can now be exerted and, using
appropriate blunt curved scissors, the
artery can be traced downwards, cutting
the adventitia over it until the first
bifurcation is reached.

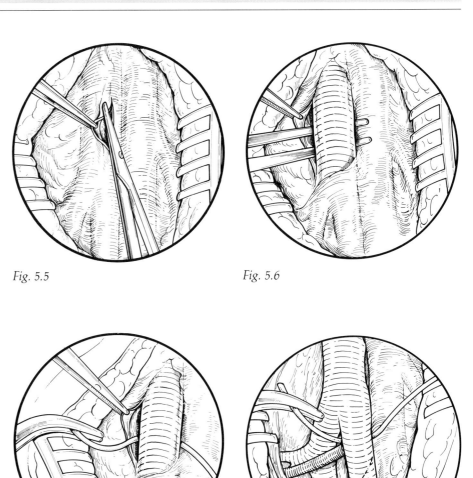

Fig. 5.5

Fig. 5.6

Fig. 5.7

Fig. 5.8

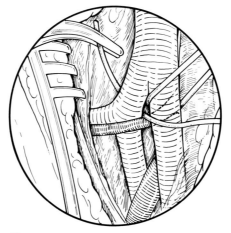

Fig. 5.9

At or before this point, a small vein will usually be encountered, this should be isolated, doubly ligated and divided. This will usually expose the first two branches which can be separately encircled by fine silastic slings (Figs 5.10, 5.11). This must be done very carefully as the vessels are extremely thin.

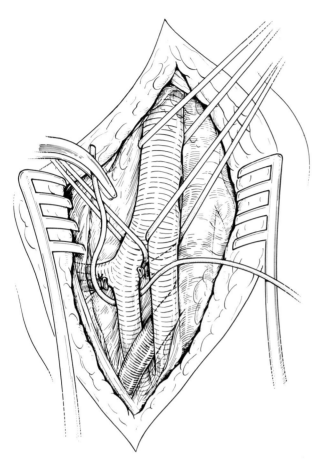

Fig. 5.10

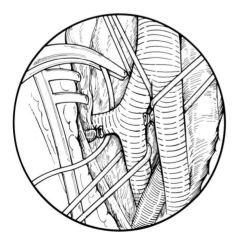

Fig. 5.11

INTRAOPERATIVE INVESTIGATIONS

At this point the significance of the profunda stenosis can be assessed by performing a papaverine test, but this is not essential and must be done carefully. A 21-gauge needle is inserted into the front of the profunda femoris artery below what is known to be the area of narrowing on the preoperative arteriogram. Be careful here because the artery is very thin and can easily be damaged. A reference needle is placed either in the common femoral artery or preferably in the radial artery. This is usually done by the anaesthetist pre-operatively. Resting pressure levels are measured and 20 mg of papaverine injected directly via the needle in the profunda femoris vessel. A fall in pressure of more than 20%, or a resting pressure

drop in excess of 10 mmHg are evidence of a severe stenosis (see p. 5). With this evidence of functional stenosis, and provided that a reasonable preoperative arteriogram shows that the rest of the profunda tree is relatively normal, no further dissection is required. If, however, further stenoses can be seen lower down the profunda femoris artery, the incision must be extended until the last stenotic area has been reached. If the picture of the distal profunda is inadequate, then an on-table arteriogram should be performed as previously described. If the dissection is to be taken more distally, it is usually necessary to follow the profunda femoris artery downwards, dividing the profunda femoris vein between ligatures (see later). Having defined the level of stenosis, the patient is given heparin (5000 units) systemically and the

common femoral artery occluded with a vascular clamp about 3 cm above the bifurcation. Other clamps are placed on the superficial femoral artery and the branches of the profunda femoris if necessary. These can, however, usually be controlled by gentle traction on the silastic slings around them. An incision is then made in the common femoral artery above the bifurcation using a scalpel with a pointed tip. Care should be taken not to cut too deeply as it is possible to perforate both walls of the vessel (Fig. 5.12). Once blood emerges from the arteriotomy, a pair of right-angled scissors is used to extend the incision in the vessel downwards and across the mouth of the profunda femoris artery (Fig. 5.13). This incision is taken as far distally as necessary to ensure that the stenosis has been completely divided (Fig. 5.14). The

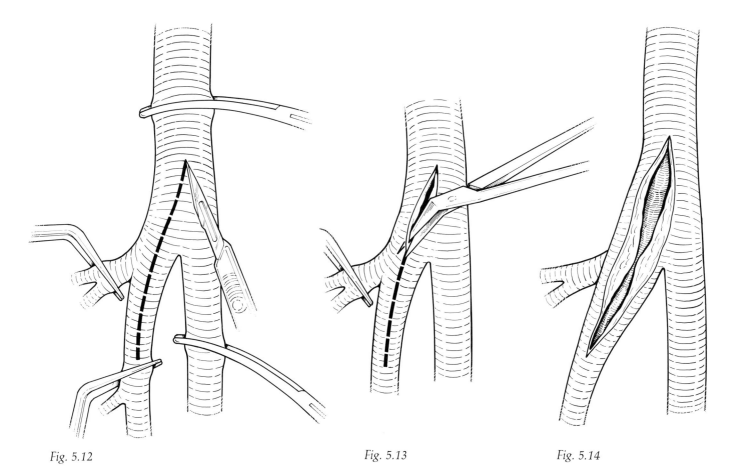

Fig. 5.12   *Fig. 5.13*   *Fig. 5.14*

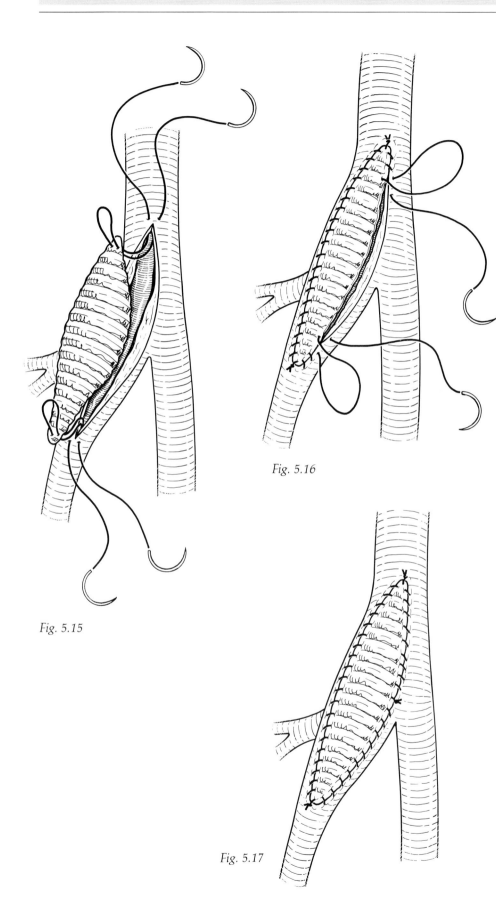

Fig. 5.15

Fig. 5.16

Fig. 5.17

vessel beyond will be wider and the intima clearly much thinner. In general, the area of atheroma causing the stenosis should not be disturbed. If, however, it is clearly ulcerated, or leaving it would produce unacceptable obstruction to flow, then it must be removed by endarterectomy (see later). Once the limits of the lesion have been reached, a suitable patch is chosen to close the defect. In general, vein is the best material to use to close the arteriotomy. If the possibility of distal reconstruction has been excluded then it is reasonable to use part of the long saphenous vein or one of its branches: a segment of a vein removed from the ankle is the best choice as it does not interfere with the rest of the vein. Alternatively, a vein can be taken from the arm. Failing this a patch of Dacron, PTFE or umbilical vein is acceptable but less than ideal. An endarterectomised segment of the blocked superficial femoral artery can also be used as an isolated patch or swung across as a flap. Whatever is used, the patch is shaped to fit the arteriotomy and sutured into place using either 5 or 6/0 double-ended monofilament nylon. Each end is first of all secured with separate stitches, ensuring that the needle passes from the inside to the outside of the artery (Fig. 5.15). Once the patch has been tied in place, one side is sutured with an over-and-over continuous stitch. This stitch is tied to its fellow once that side of the anastomosis is completed. The remaining side is completed with a similar technique (Fig. 5.16), using both needles in turn and finishing in the middle of the second side (Fig. 5.17). Before the last stitch is tied, the clamps are released to ensure adequate back bleeding from both branches of the profunda femoris, also forward bleeding from the femoral artery. Finally, the clamps are released, starting with the distal one first.

ASSESSMENT OF THE PROCEDURE

A needle should once again be inserted distal to the patch and the papaverine test repeated. If a successful reconstruction has been achieved, then the pressure drop seen preoperatively should be abolished. However, it is not usually necessary to do this as damage to the vessel can occur very easily.

EXTENDED PROFUNDAPLASTY

Extension of the procedure well down the thigh was favoured by Cotton,[3] but is not usually necessary unless there are multiple stenoses in the vessel or a long occlusion. If it proves necessary to extend the exposure of the vessels beyond the first bifurcation, the profunda femoris vein, which will be seen crossing the artery from the lateral to the medial side, has to be divided (Fig. 5.18). This is a large structure and needs to be carefully tied, preferably with a transfixing suture, or oversewn. Once this vein has been ligated and divided, access to the vessel where it passes deep to adductor longus and vastus medialis becomes easier (Fig. 5.19). Again, by appropriate retraction and division of the muscular tissue in front of the artery, it is possible to follow it for as long as is necessary and go beyond the area of the last stricture (Fig. 5.20). Once this has been done, then patching it proceeds in the same way as already described for a limited profundaplasty (Fig. 5.21). However, for distal reconstructions vein should probably always be used.

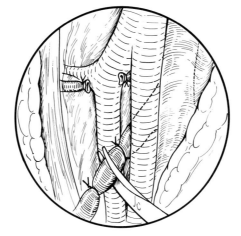

Fig. 5.18

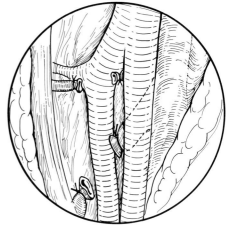

Fig. 5.19

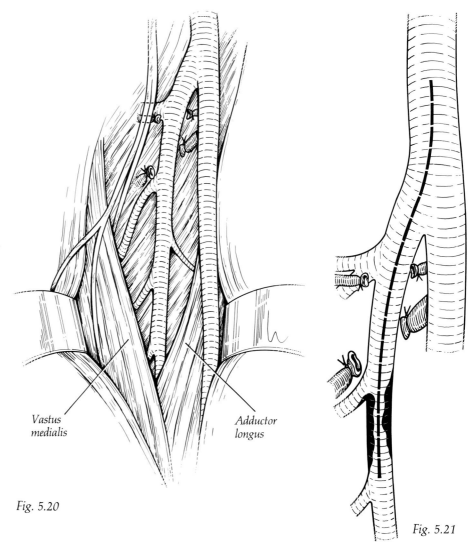

Vastus medialis

Adductor longus

Fig. 5.20

Fig. 5.21

ENDARTERECTOMY

An endarterectomy should not be performed if it can be avoided. However, if the area of atheroma at the origin of the profunda femoris artery is extensive with a clearly defined lumen beyond, then a localised endarterectomy should be carefully performed (Fig. 5.22). In order to do this, establish the line of cleavage between the atheroma and the muscular wall of the artery—this can usually be easily seen as a potential space—and using the blunt end of a blunt dissector, such as a Watson Cheyne dissector, it is possible to separate the atheromatous plaque by gentle dissection (Fig. 5.23). Once the dissection has proceeded into the common femoral artery, the plaque is cut across obliquely, ignoring the origin of the superficial femoral which is usually blocked in these cases (Fig. 5.24). Distally, the atheromatous plaque is dissected free until an area is reached where it is reasonably thin.

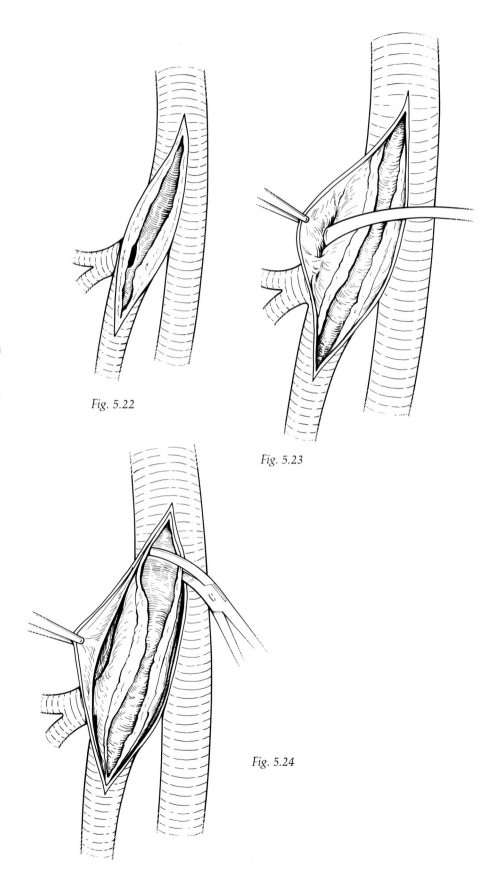

Fig. 5.22

Fig. 5.23

Fig. 5.24

At this point, the atheroma is again cut obliquely so as to present a relatively narrow face to the onflowing blood (Fig. 5.25). If the thickening continues, then it must be followed as far as necessary, even by extending the incision and the arteriotomy as for deep extended profundaplasty. Because it is likely that, once the endarterectomy has started, it will need to be continued for much longer than the operator at first envisaged, it should not be done lightly. Once the plaque has been removed the distal flap should be secured, if necessary, by suturing interrupted 7–8/0 Prolene stitches to the arterial wall, the knot being tied on the outside (Fig. 5.26). These are inserted circumferentially. Once this has been done, the vessel is patched as described previously.

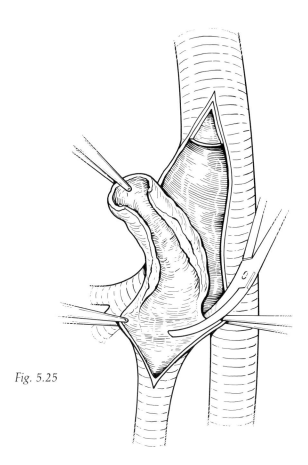

Fig. 5.25

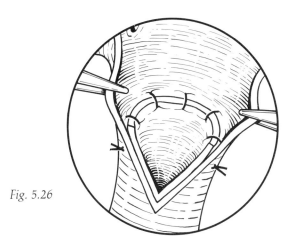

Fig. 5.26

DISTAL APPROACH TO THE PROFUNDA FEMORIS

Sometimes the profunda femoris artery is difficult or impossible to approach because of previous surgery. Under these circumstances the more distal, probably undisturbed, portion of the profunda femoris can be approached directly without exposure of the common or superficial femoral artery and the proximal zone of the profunda.[4] The middle and distal zones of the vessel can be exposed by an incision passing along the medial border of the sartorius muscle, which is then pushed laterally, or the lateral border with the muscle pushed medially. The adductor longus muscle lies directly behind the sartorius and the profunda is approached by dissection in front of, or behind it (Fig. 5.27). There is usually a dense fibrous sheet from the adductor magnus to the vastus medialis and the profunda femoris artery can usually be felt behind this as a longitudinal cord-like structure, which is approached after division of this connective tissue sheet.

Sometimes in this situation the profunda is not patent until its distal end. In this case, a reversed vein graft from the femoral artery to the distal patent profunda may be a better option than a very long vein patch (Fig. 5.28).

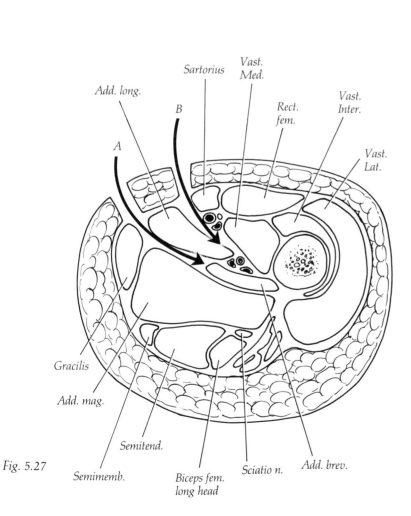

Add. long.

B

A

Sartorius

*Vast.
Med.*

*Rect.
fem.*

*Vast.
Inter.*

*Vast.
Lat.*

Gracilis

Add. mag.

Semitend.

Semimemb.

*Biceps fem.
long head*

Sciatio n.

Add. brev.

Fig. 5.27

Fig. 5.28

OTHER METHODS OF PATCHING THE PROFUNDA

The use of long saphenous or arm vein has already been mentioned. Other methods can also be considered which involve using the usually blocked superficial femoral artery. For example, a piece of this can be excised, the atheroma removed by endarterectomy and the vessel used for a patch (Fig. 5.29). The profunda stenosis, particularly if it is short, can be widened by stitching the origins of the superficial femoral and profunda femoris together (Figs 5.30, 5.31 and 5.32). Lastly, the superficial femoral artery can be divided as in Figures 5.33 and 5.34 and the vessel swung over to act as a patch.

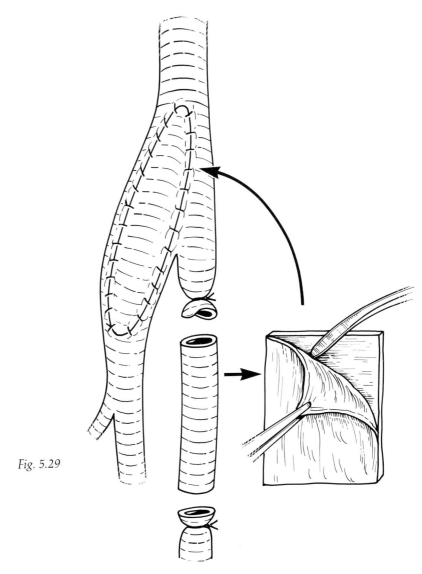

Fig. 5.29

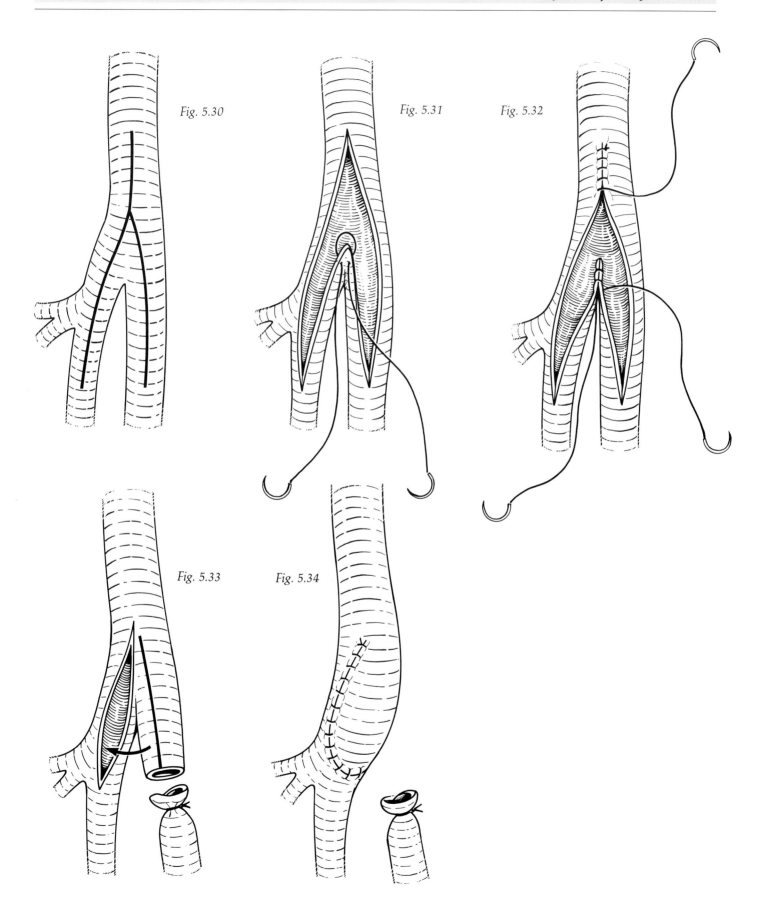

Fig. 5.30

Fig. 5.31

Fig. 5.32

Fig. 5.33

Fig. 5.34

PROFUNDAPLASTY WITH PROXIMAL RECONSTRUCTION

The most common reason for doing a profundaplasty is when the distal end of a bifurcated or iliofemoral graft is stitched across the origin of the profunda femoris artery. Occasionally it may be necessary, or seem appropriate, to carry out an iliofemoral endarterectomy and patch the entire segment by carrying it into the profunda. In that event, the iliac artery must, of course, be exposed above the inguinal ligament as described later for iliofemoral grafting via the obturator foramen (p. 78).

IMPORTANT POINTS IN THE OPERATION

1.   Has the arteriotomy been extended far enough down the vessel? If you are unsure, check the preoperative arteriograms or do more on the table.
2.   Is a local endarterectomy necessary? If possible do not do one. Having opened the profunda across its origin, try and picture what it would look like with a patch in place. When patched, if the atheroma does not encroach significantly on the lumen, i.e. less than 50%, leave it alone. If you are unhappy, then do an endarterectomy.
3.   If an endarterectomy is done how far distally should you go? Take the endarterectomy to the next reasonable area of intima and then cut this obliquely and sew it down to prevent dissection later. Make sure that the patch extends well beyond where you have stopped the endarterectomy.
4.   What should you use for a patch? Use vein if possible, but only if it is readily available and, if using a piece of saphenous vein, it is not going to jeopardise a future operation (i.e. take it from the ankle or arm), otherwise use a piece of woven Dacron or endarterectomised femoral artery. For very distal procedures vein must be used.

POSTOPERATIVE CARE

There are no special points to bear in mind. The pulses will not be palpable, but success should be obvious by a better capillary return to the foot and possibly increased ankle pressures. Bleeding should, of course, be remembered, particularly as the patient's heparinisation will not usually have been reversed after surgery unless there are specific indications for doing so. A fine suction drain should be inserted for 24 hours.

COMPLICATIONS

Lymphatic leakage
This can occur and be a problem, usually in a minority of cases, particularly if potential lymphatic channels have not been properly ligated. If it does occur, the patient's antibiotic therapy should be continued and the wound kept clean and covered. It should stop spontaneously.

Haemorrhage
Always a possibility following vascular surgery. Should it occur, the patient will need to be taken back to theatre and the appropriate steps taken to stop it.

Infection
If artificial materials are used then infection is a possibility. If it occurs, it will usually not respond to antibiotic therapy and secondary haemorrhage will inevitably result. In that event the graft will have to be removed and replaced, if possible with non-synthetic materials such as vein, which will be very difficult. Even then it is likely that deterioration of the limb will occur and possibly result in an amputation, particularly in this sort of case where other options are few.

Thrombosis
If the profunda thromboses, the femoral pulse will disappear as the profunda femoris is the only run-off vessel. In addition, the circulation to the foot may deteriorate. If this happens, then the patient should be returned to theatre and one edge of the patch opened, the inside of the vessel inspected thoroughly and the thrombus removed completely with a Fogarty catheter. If good back bleeding is present, the patient should be heparinised with a single dose of systemic heparin and the wound closed. These vessels do not usually thrombose unless there is a very poor run off.

RESULTS

If this procedure is used in the kind of case mentioned above, then the results can be good.[5] If an extended profundaplasty is performed without an obvious stenosis and in the absence of the criteria set out above, the results are not particularly good and the patient may eventually require an amputation because of a lack of improvement to the circulation.

REFERENCES

1   Natali J 1962 Profunda femoris reconstruction. Journal de Chirurgie 83:
     4–12
2   Martin P, Renwick S, Stevenson C 1968 On the surgery of the
     profundafemoris artery. British Journal of Surgery 55: 539–542
3   Thomas M H, Quick C R C, Cotton L T 1977 Doppler ultrasound in the
     functional assessment of deep femoral angioplasty. British Journal of
     Surgery 64: 368–372
4   Nunez A A, Veith F J, Collier P, Ascer E, White-Flores S, Gupta S 1988
     Direct approaches to the distal portions of the deep femoral artery
     for limb salvage. Journal of Vascular Surgery 8: 576–581
5   Hill D A, Jamieson C W 1979 The results of surgical reconstruction of
     the profundafemoris artery in the treatment of rest pain and
     gangrene. British Journal of Surgery 64: 362–368

Chapter 6

Aneurysms of the femoral artery

Introduction

Aneurysms of the femoral artery can either be true aneurysms, which are usually fusiform in nature, or they can be anastomotic or false.

TRUE ANEURYSMS

These lesions are relatively uncommon and often found as an incidental finding in elderly patients, usually male. However, they can occur with aortic or popliteal aneurysms, which should always be looked for in such patients.[1] They are frequently bilateral and can involve the profunda femoris artery as well as the common and superficial femoral artery.

Presentation and indications for surgery

They are usually asymptomatic and gradually enlarge with time, but can rupture[2] or lead to distal embolisation. Occasionally they can thrombose and present with an acutely ischaemic limb, or cause local pressure symptoms or a swollen limb.[3] If they present in an elderly, unfit patient they should be left alone and observed. If, however, they appear to be enlarging or producing symptoms from local pressure, leg swelling or embolisation, they should be dealt with surgically.

Preoperative investigations

The diagnosis is usually obvious, but if it is not, ultrasound will be helpful. Arteriography will show the profunda anatomy but is not mandatory.

Operative technique

The patient should be given antibiotic cover as already described in Chapter 1, because the groin in particular is an area where infection can easily occur. The patient is placed in the supine position under general anaesthesia, although spinal anaesthesia can be adequate. Because of the possibility that access to the iliac and femoral arteries may be necessary, the patient's skin should be prepared to allow access to these vessels. The initial incision should be an oblique or vertical one over the aneurysm, as already described for exposure of the femoral artery on page 48. The deep fascia is carefully dissected with a pair of atraumatic scissors until the wall of the sac is encountered (Fig. 6.1). At this point it is important to decide the limits of the lesion in order that proximal control can be gained. If the common femoral artery appears to be normal, then it should be encircled with a silastic sling. However, if there is any doubt about the extent of the lesion, it is safer to make a second oblique incision above the inguinal ligament, cut through the external, internal oblique and transversus muscles and approach the iliac artery in the

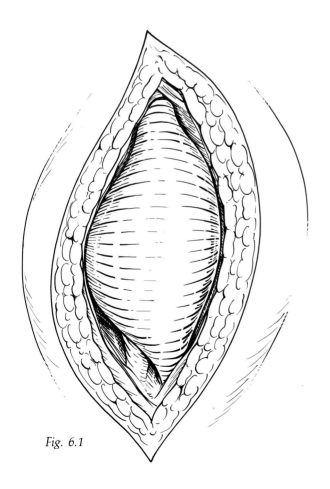

Fig. 6.1

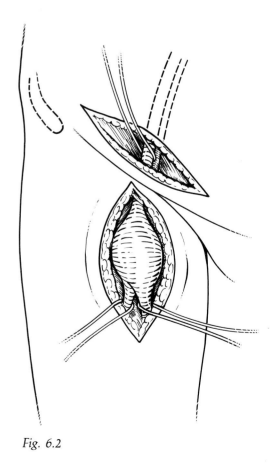

Fig. 6.2

retroperitoneal plane immediately above the inguinal ligament. At this point it can be dissected free and controlled with a silastic sling (Fig. 6.2). This manoeuvre takes a few minutes and allows complete and safe control avoiding later haemorrhage. Once proximal control has been achieved by either of these two means, the rest of the sac is then dissected free, the aim being to gain control of the superficial femoral and profunda femoris arteries (Fig. 6.2). Care should be taken not to rupture the sac as the wall can be quite thin in places and gentle sharp dissection is the best technique to use. If the profunda femoris and superficial femoral arteries are not involved in the

aneurysm these can be encircled and controlled with silastic slings (Fig. 6.2). Make sure that the profunda is dissected down to the first bifurcation and each branch controlled as for profundaplasty (p. 48). If they are involved in the aneurysm, however, this might be difficult, particularly in the case of the profunda femoris artery. Once control has been achieved, what is done next will depend upon the findings.

Aneurysm limited to the common femoral artery
In this situation the common femoral above the sac, the profunda femoris and superficial femoral are clamped after heparinising the patient. The sac is

opened longitudinally (Fig. 6.3) and the gap bridged with a small (12 mm) woven Dacron graft, which is inserted between the common femoral and its bifurcation (Fig. 6.4). The vessels should be divided completely across if this proves possible and an end-to-end anastomosis performed above and below to each vessel, as described on page 28. If the vessels are very small it is preferable to use saphenous vein.

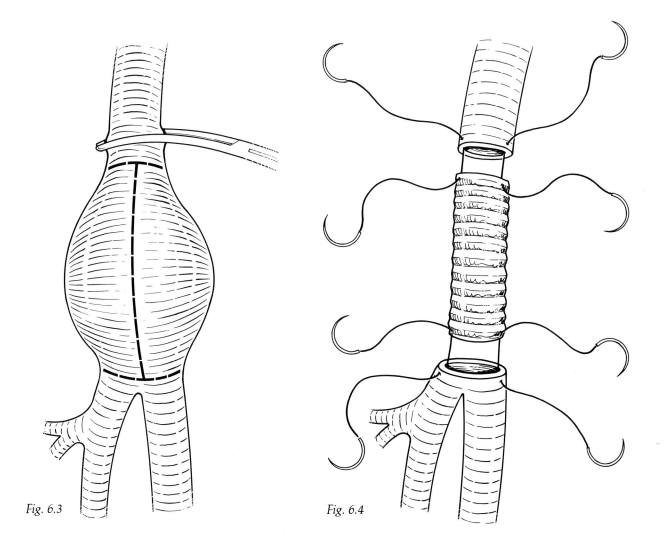

Fig. 6.3

Fig. 6.4

Aneurysm involving the profunda femoris, superficial femoral and common femoral arteries

If possible, the vessels above and below the sac are controlled, clamped and the sac opened longitudinally (Fig. 6.5), the vessels divided and a 12 mm woven Dacron graft inserted (Fig. 6.6). If the vessels are small, it is best to use the saphenous vein, particularly if a branched segment is available. In a situation where the profunda femoris cannot be easily controlled, the best plan is to clamp the common femoral artery above the sac, control the superficial femoral artery, open the sac and then pass a Fogarty catheter (no. 2 or 3) into the profunda femoris orifice, which will be bleeding freely.

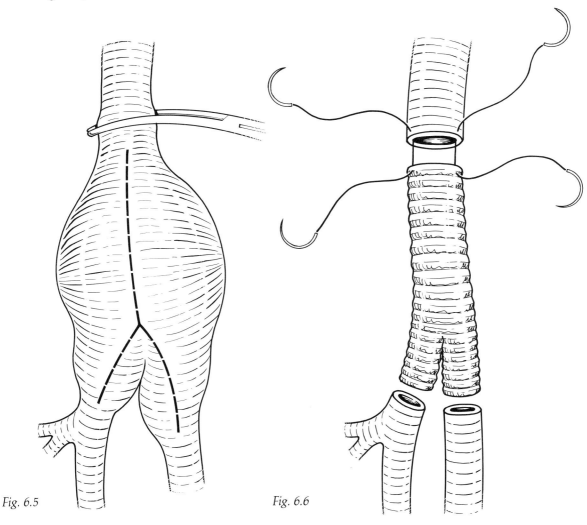

Fig. 6.5   *Fig. 6.6*

The catheter is attached to a three-way tap and, by inflating the balloon, the Fogarty catheter can be used to control retrograde flow from the profunda femoris (Fig. 6.7). Once control is achieved as before it will usually be best to stitch the bifurcated graft (12 mm) separately to the superficial femoral artery, if it is patent, and the profunda femoris. If this method of control is to be used it is best, but not essential, to pass the Fogarty catheter down one limb of the bifurcated graft and complete the distal

anastomoses first. The Fogarty catheter can then be removed, the graft clamped and the proximal anastomosis constructed without difficulty (Fig. 6.7). Once again, the proximal anastomosis is performed after dividing the femoral artery, as already described on page 30. The distal anastomosis is done in a similar fashion if the vessels can be divided (Fig. 6.7). If the profunda, in particular, cannot be completely divided the graft should be stitched to the orifice with the back wall intact, starting with the back wall first as in an aortic

aneurysm (Fig. 6.16). If the sac is large enough it should be sutured over the graft, if not it should be excised carefully and the groin wound drained for 24 hours.

Additional procedures
If a patient has an associated occlusion of the superficial femoral artery with a poor profunda, it may be necessary to place an additional graft down to the popliteal artery either above or below the knee. If this is the case then the graft, which is usually PTFE or autologous vein, should be sutured end-to-side with the graft which has already been inserted to replace the aneurysms above (Fig. 6.8) and the popliteal artery below.

Problems in the operation
The main problem, if the sac involves the profunda femoris artery, is control of this vessel. The best technique is to use a Fogarty catheter to obstruct the orifice, which will prevent bleeding and allow this anastomosis to take place. If the vessels are particularly friable it might be necessary to stitch a piece of vein around the orifice prior to anastomosing this graft as for the Miller cuff (p. 173). Rough handling of the sac can cause rupture before full control is achieved, which is why proximal control should always be achieved before a full dissection is undertaken. If a rupture then occurs, and cannot easily be controlled by pressure, the sac should be opened and the profunda and superficial femoral arteries occluded with a Fogarty catheter, as already described.

Results
The results of surgery for aneurysms of the femoral artery are excellent, especially for asymptomatic lesions, and once they have been dealt with do not usually recur.[4]

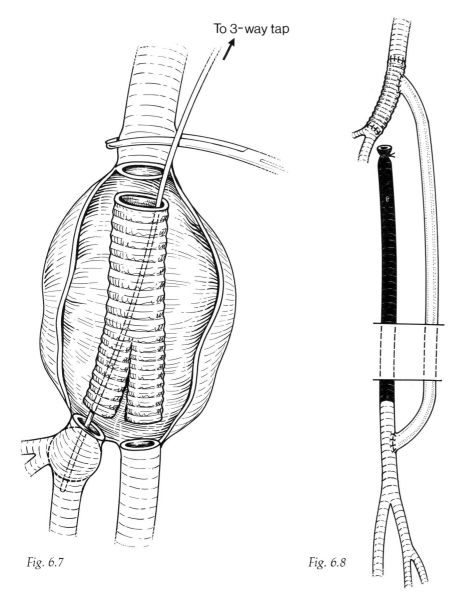

To 3-way tap

Fig. 6.7

Fig. 6.8

ANASTOMOTIC ANEURYSMS

These lesions will occur in any population of patients who have had a previous grafting procedure to the femoral artery (Fig. 6.9). The incidence is 1–5% in such a population, being commonest in patients who have had aortobifemoral grafts.[5,6] The cause of these aneurysms is uncertain and may be due to degeneration of suture material or to excessive thinning of the vessels at the anastomosis due to an endarterectomy being performed at the time of surgery. The aneurysm can either be infected, in which case it will present with discharge or bleeding at the groin and should be dealt with as described in Chapter 7 for iliofemoral lesions, where a bypass through the obturator foramen will be necessary to solve the problem. Most frequently, however, they are not infected and gradually increase in size without symptoms. They are prone to rupture or erosion through the skin and should usually be dealt with surgically.

Operation
The patient will again need antibiotic cover and is placed in the supine position. The groin is cleaned as before to include the lower abdomen and the leg down to the midcalf. For these aneurysms it is usually wise to expose the graft first, just above the inguinal ligament, through a separate incision placed obliquely and passing through the muscles of the abdominal wall (Fig. 6.10). The graft is approached retroperitoneally and if it is of woven Dacron can easily be dissected free after incising the fibrous capsule around it, as described for iliofemoral grafts on page 79. It is then encircled and controlled with a silastic sling.

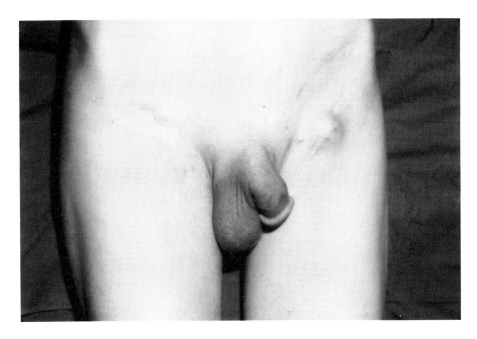

Fig. 6.9
A left false aneurysm in a patient with a previously inserted bifurcated graft. The right side is normal.

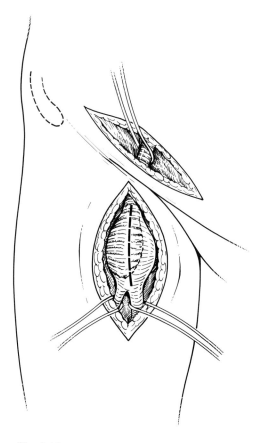

Fig. 6.10

Once this has been done, the aneurysm itself is exposed through a vertical incision as for a true aneurysm. The skin and deep fascia are separated from the sac using sharp dissection and, if possible, the profunda femoris and superficial femoral arteries are exposed and controlled with silastic slings (Fig. 6.11). This may be difficult because of the previous surgery and sharp dissection is usually essential in order to achieve a plane of cleavage—sometimes a scalpel has to be used for this purpose. If control of the superficial femoral and profunda femoris arteries can be achieved, the patient is heparinised, the graft clamped proximally and a vertical incision made in the sac (Fig. 6.10), which will consist mostly of the graft where it is separated from the arterial wall. In most cases it is then possible to excise the redundant part of the graft from the artery and cut back some of the arterial wall leaving a reasonable orifice to which a new graft can be stitched (Fig. 6.12).

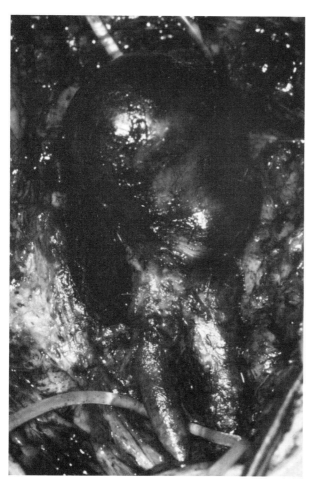

Fig. 6.11
False aneurysm after dissection showing the sac with the profunda and superficial femoral arteries dissected out.

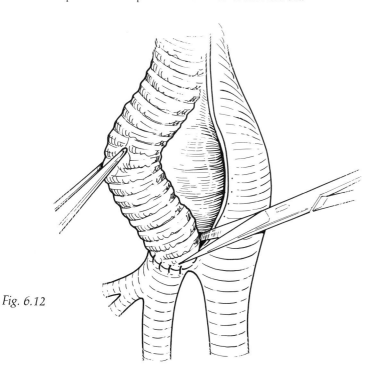

Fig. 6.12

Proximally the graft is divided and a new piece anastomosed to it using an end to end technique as described on page 28. The lower end is then stitched to the opening in the femoral artery using an end-to-side technique as described on page 31. Dacron (8–10 mm), either woven or knitted, is best for this situation (Fig. 6.13). If it is not possible to control the profunda femoris and superficial femoral artery because of fibrosis, then control can be achieved as already described for a true aneurysm.

The sac is opened, after proximal clamping, and retrograde bleeding from the superficial and profunda femoris arteries stopped by inserting a Fogarty catheter attached to a three-way tap and inflating the balloon (Fig. 6.14). This is usually only necessary for the profunda femoris as the superficial femoral can usually be controlled, or is often blocked. After this has been done, the graft can be interposed between the existing divided graft proximally using an end-to-end anastomosis and distally sutured to the orifice of the profunda

femoris artery and the superficial femoral if it is patent. Again, a small bifurcated graft is often useful for this part of the operation. If a Fogarty catheter has been used to control bleeding, the catheter should again be passed through the graft before the balloon is inflated (Fig. 6.7) and the lower anastomosis constructed without dividing the back wall of the profunda.

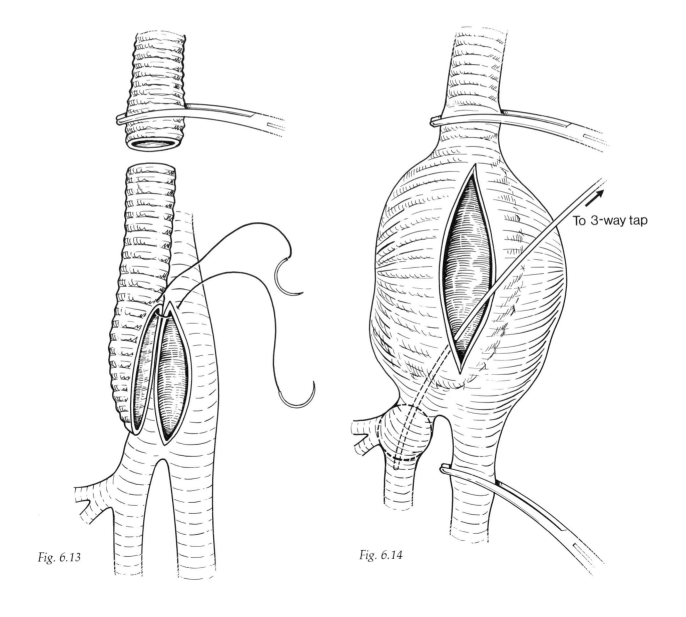

To 3-way tap

Fig. 6.13   *Fig. 6.14*

After the initial suture has been inserted (Fig. 6.15), it is tied and one stitch passed to the left behind the graft. The anastomosis is now completed from the middle of the back wall, passing outwards with each stitch (Fig. 6.16). Prolene (50 or 60) is usually the best material to use for both of these anastomoses. If the profunda femoris is difficult to see and a Fogarty catheter has been used to control back bleeding, it may not be possible to divide the vessel completely. If this is the case, and especially if the vessel is friable, it is best to use a piece of reversed saphenous vein if this is available.

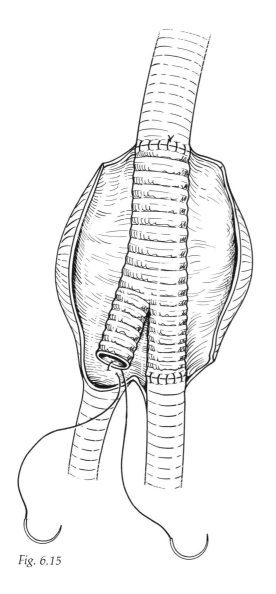

Fig. 6.15

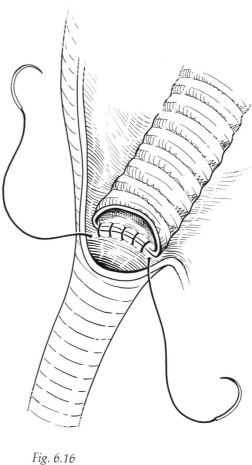

Fig. 6.16

If it is not, then PTFE might be appropriate, the lower end being attached to the profunda femoris artery using an interposed Miller collar of autologous vein (Fig. 6.17), as described for femorodistal grafts on page 173. The collar is stitched to the profunda in exactly the same way as shown in Figure 6.15. The superficial femoral artery is often occluded and requires no attention, but if the profunda femoris is compromised it may be necessary to insert an additional femoropopliteal graft to the above- or below-knee popliteal artery, stitching the top end of the graft onto the interposed segment and the lower end to the appropriate part of the popliteal artery (Fig. 6.8), as described for the femoropopliteal grafting on page 108.

Results

The results of this type of procedure are usually good if infection is not present.[7,8] If the arterial wall is not cut back sufficiently, however, the lesion can recur. If there is any doubt about the usefulness of the arterial wall, then it should be excised completely and a straight or bifurcated graft sewn to both profunda and superficial femoral artery separately.

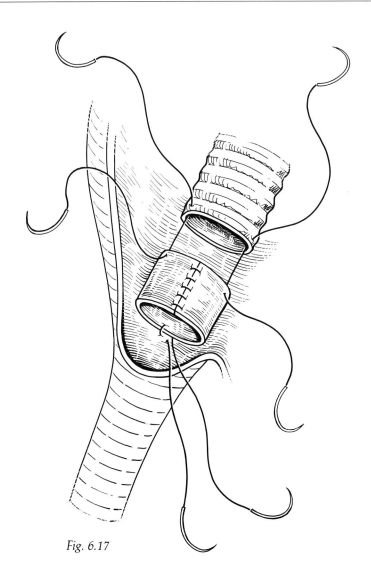

Fig. 6.17

FALSE ANEURYSM

A false aneurysm usually occurs after inadequate pressure is placed on the femoral artery following an angiogram or angioplasty. Blood emerges from the opening in the artery and collects around the vessel, causing a swelling which gradually enlarges and becomes pulsatile. In any patient in whom there is a swelling following such a procedure, a false aneurysm should be considered as the most likely cause. The lesion is easily dealt with by a vertical incision over the artery which can then be controlled proximally by exposing the common femoral artery and encircling it with a sling. Once this has been done, the vessel is clamped and the false aneurysm opened without undue dissection. The blood clot is removed and a small opening will usually be seen in the front of the femoral artery where the catheter, which caused the lesion, entered. This can be dealt with by one or two 5/0 sutures to close the hole. Thereafter, the clamp can be released resolving the problem; the wound should be drained for 24 hours.

REFERENCES

1   Graham L, Zelenock G, Whitehouse W et al 1980 Clinical significance of arteriosclerotic femoral artery aneurysms. Archives of Surgery 115: 502–507
2   Baird R J, Garry J F, Kellam J et al 1977 Arteriosclerotic femoral artery aneurysms. Canadian Medical Association Journal 117: 1306–1307
3   Catler B S, Darling R C 1973 Surgical management of arteriosclerotic femoral aneurysms. Surgery 74: 764–773
4   Adiseshia M, Bailey D A 1977 Aneurysms of the femoral artery. British Journal of Surgery 64: 174–176
5   Courbier R, Larranga J 1982 Natural history and management of anastomotic aneurysms. In: Bergen J J, Yao J S T (eds) Aneurysms. Grune and Stratton, New York, pp 567–580
6   Szilagyi D I, Elliott J P, Smith R F, Reddy D J, Mcpharlin M 1986 A 30-year study of the reconstructive surgical treatment of aortoiliac occlusive disease. Journal of Vascular Surgery 3: 421–436
7   Hollier L H, Batson R C, Cotton I 1981 Femoral anastomotic aneurysms. Surgery 191: 715–720
8   Berridge D C, Earnshaw J J, Makin G S, Hopkinson B R 1988 A 10-year review of false aneurysms in Nottingham. Annals of the Royal College of Surgeons of England 70: 253–256

Chapter 7

Iliopopliteal grafts

Introduction

Iliopopliteal grafts are rarely required except when there is a proximal block and the profunda femoris artery is inoperable—a rare situation. They are needed, however, when serious sepsis occurs in the groin in association with a vascular anastomosis. In this situation the graft has to be inserted in the extra-anatomic position, which will be described shortly. If sepsis is not a problem, PTFE or Dacron can be taken from the common iliac artery above (end-to-side), tunnelled under the inguinal ligament and sutured to the popliteal artery above the knee. The iliac artery can be exposed, as will be described for extra-anatomic procedures, and the above-knee popliteal artery as for above knee femoropopliteal grafting (p. 108). It is usually necessary to make a third small incision below the inguinal ligament to facilitate tunnelling of the graft.

ILIOPOPLITEAL GRAFTS VIA THE OBTURATOR FORAMEN

The indication for this procedure is sepsis in the groin, with the need for a bypass procedure between the aorta and the lower limb. A common indication would be if sepsis occurred in one limb of a bifurcated or unilateral iliofemoral graft, with secondary haemorrhage or exposure of the graft material.[1,2] In this situation, the existing graft has to be removed and replaced with a new piece which can circumvent the infected area. Another indication would be in a patient with superficial groin sepsis, such as intertrigo, where an urgent aortofemoral procedure is necessary.

PREPARATION FOR THE OPERATION

For this operation to succeed the patient has to have a patent femoral artery below the area of sepsis. Revascularisation of the profunda cannot be relied upon because it is usually in the middle of a septic area and, if a previous graft has been inserted, it is usually involved in that anastomosis. An adequate arteriogram is therefore essential depicting the vessels from the groin downwards. If there is no satisfactory and continuous run-off into the lower leg and foot, then the operation will probably fail. The patient has to be prepared adequately beforehand and a course of wide-spectrum antibiotics, which will cover all eventualities, should be started several days before the procedure is planned. A good combination is gentamicin, flucloxacillin and metronidazole. The infected groin area should be covered in iodine-soaked swabs (Fig. 7.1) and the patient's abdomen and lower leg should be similarly cleaned daily.

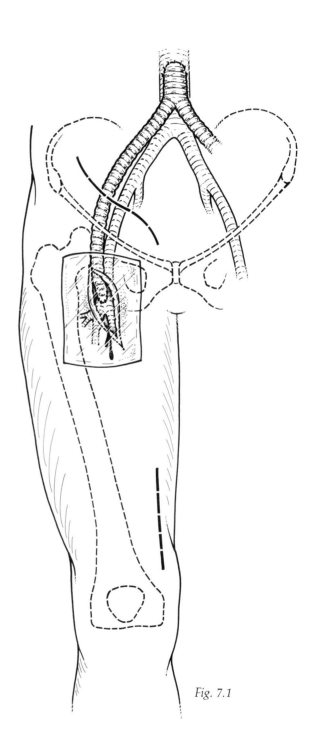

Fig. 7.1

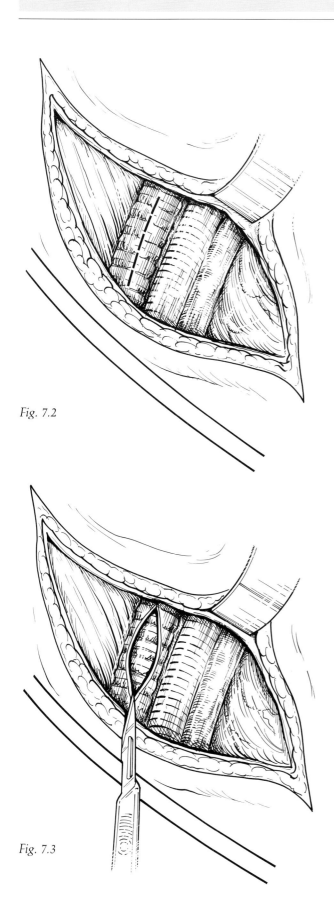

Fig. 7.2

Fig. 7.3

PROCEDURE

The patient is placed in the prone position and the exposed graft in the groin covered with an iodine-soaked swab and then a layer of transparent adhesive material to exclude it from the operative field. The rest of the operation site is then cleaned again with an appropriate alcohol-containing solution, iodine with alcohol is best.[1]

The graft is exposed above the inguinal ligament using an oblique incision, which passes through the external and internal oblique muscles and then the transversus abdominus developing in the extraperitoneal plane (Fig. 7.2). If the peritoneum is adherent, as it often is, then it may be necessary to enter the peritoneal cavity to expose the existing graft. If woven Dacron has been used, it can usually easily be exposed by sharp dissection using a scalpel to cut down onto the graft itself. Knitted Dacron causes more problems because of tissue ingrowth. The scalpel will usually pass through the thick capsule surrounding the graft, but the graft material itself (Fig. 7.3) is usually free from this capsule and can be encircled easily with a curved forcep (Fig. 7.4). One or two silastic slings should then be placed around the graft, thus gaining adequate proximal control.

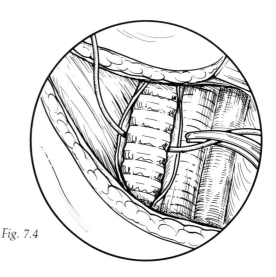

Fig. 7.4

At this point the peritoneum is
stripped further upwards to expose
the internal iliac artery and, using
the finger to pass down over the
pubic symphysis, the obturator
membrane is felt (Fig. 7.5). Having felt
it, a small incision is made in the fascia
overlying the obturator muscle, taking
care to avoid any accessory vessels.
This is difficult and good retraction is
essential (Fig. 7.6). The femoral artery
above the knee is then exposed through
a medial incision, as described for
femoropopliteal bypass above the knee
(p. 108).

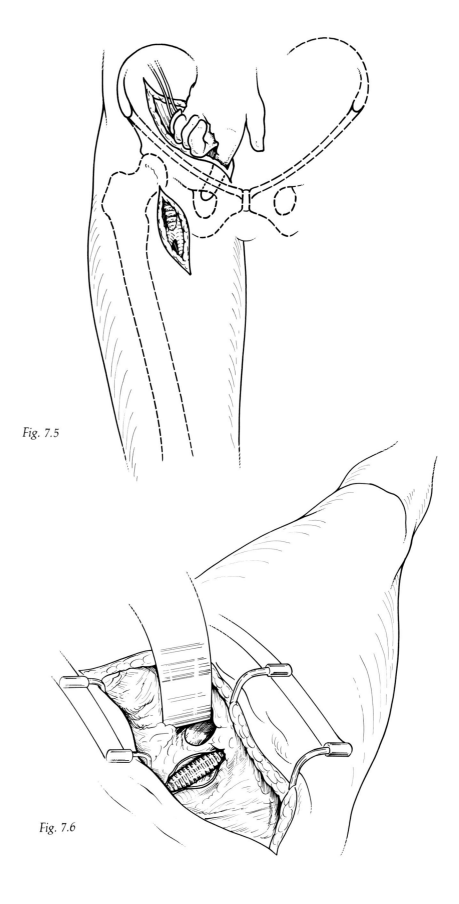

Fig. 7.5

Fig. 7.6

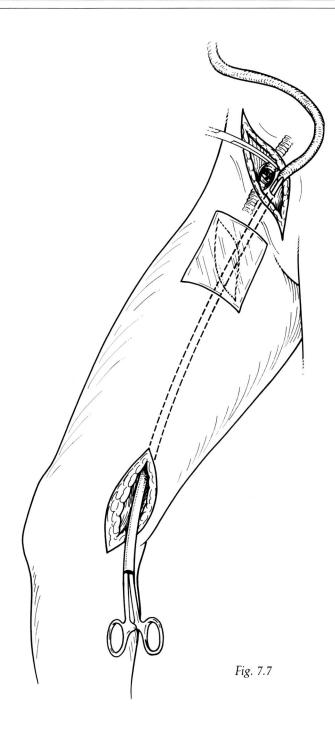

Fig. 7.7

The vessel is controlled with silastic slings and a tunnelling device then passed upwards deep inside the leg (Fig. 7.7). If a finger is placed over the obturator membrane using the left hand (for the right leg), the right hand can then be used to push the tunnelling instrument deep inside the adductor muscles up towards the membrane. The depth must be judged approximately, but the end of the tunneller must be kept away from the infected groin. Gradually, by a process of gentle pressure, the end of the tunneller will be felt against the obturator membrane. This can be made easier by slight flexion of the knee and hip. An incision is then made over it, or the existing incision enlarged and the tunneller pushed through the membrane. The new graft, which will usually be a piece of straight 10 mm woven Dacron or PTFE, is grasped through the tunneller and pulled down into the lower femoral incision.

The tunneller is removed and the distal anastomosis completed as for femoropopliteal graft (p. 108) (Fig. 7.8) using two layers of continuous 5/0 Prolene. As usual, before the final suture is inserted adequate back-bleeding is confirmed. A vascular clamp is then placed across the lower end of the graft, the upper end being pulled gently with the leg straightened until the graft is straight and the tension correct. The old graft, which had been previously exposed in an area free of infection, is then clamped, divided and the lower end ligated. An end-to-end anastomosis is then performed (Fig. 7.9) between the graft passing through the obturator membrane and the remainder of the right limb of the old bifurcated graft. Before starting the anastomosis, the clamp should be released to make sure that good proximal bleeding occurs and there is no debris within the graft. Again, double-ended continuous 5/0 Prolene is used for the anastomosis and there is usually sufficient room to complete the anterior layer and then rotate the grafts to complete the posterior layer (see p. 28).

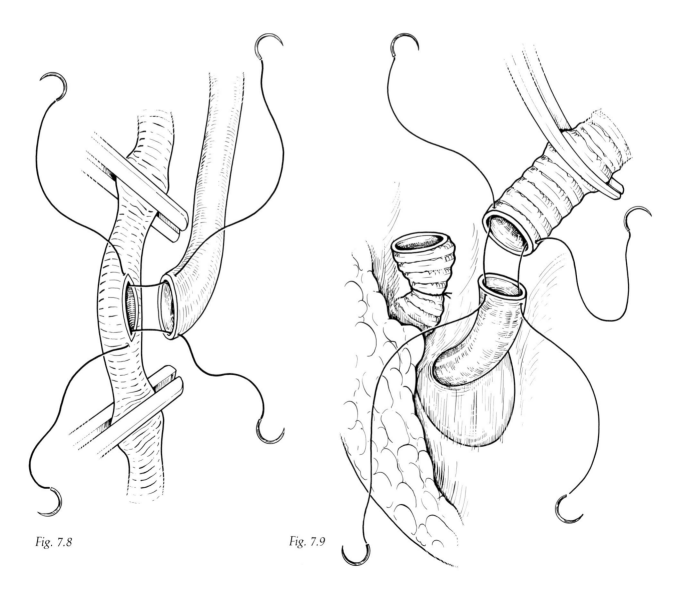

Fig. 7.8   *Fig. 7.9*

Both clamps are then released and
blood is allowed to flow down
the new graft into the lower
limb (Fig. 7.10). Success is assessed
by palpatation below the distal
anastomosis and an on-table
arteriogram is then performed to assess
the distal anastomosis and run-off. This
can be done by placing a needle into the
graft at the iliac incision, clamping it
proximally and injecting contrast (see
p. 16). If all is well, then both wounds
are closed and covered in a watertight
dressing (Fig. 7.11).

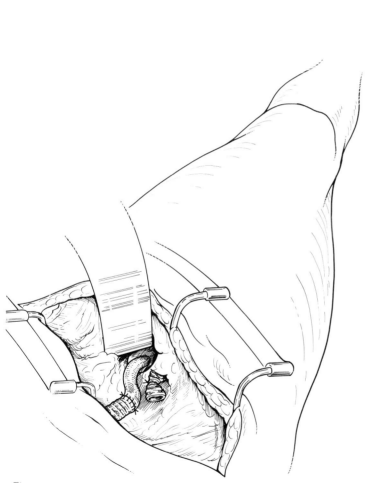

Fig. 7.10

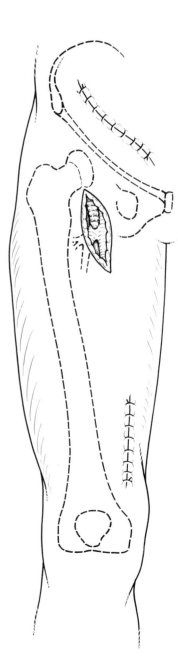

Fig. 7.11

Attention is now directed to the infected groin wound. The adhesive material is removed and the iodine-soaked pack likewise discarded. The graft is dissected distally until the profunda femoris and superficial femoral arteries have been found. This is difficult and sharp dissection with scissors or scalpel is necessary. Obvious pulsation will be present in all of these vessels from retrograde filling. Once the profunda femoris and superficial femoral have been identified they are ligated, or controlled with slings, and the graft removed by grasping it firmly with a pair of artery forceps and dividing its anastomosis with the artery (Fig. 7.12). Once the distal anastomosis has been freed, gentle downward traction on the graft will allow it to be completely removed (Fig. 7.13). This will leave a defect in the common femoral artery and profunda femoris, which can usually be oversewn, although if this is not possible the vessels are ligated (as also shown in Fig. 7.13). Finally, the groin wound is oversewn, if this proves possible, and covered in a waterproof dressing. The final position of the ilio-femoral graft and closed wounds is shown inset (Fig. 7.14).

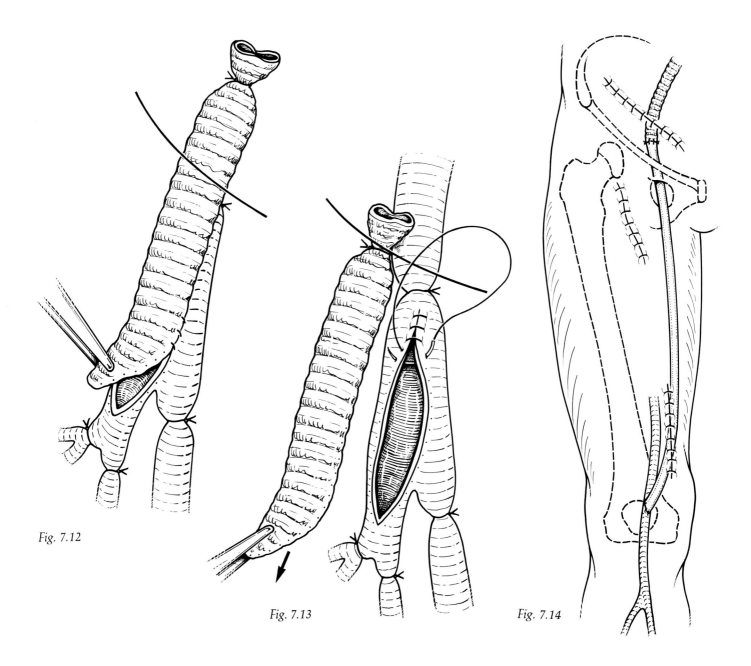

Fig. 7.12

Fig. 7.13

Fig. 7.14

PROBLEMS DURING THE OPERATION

The procedure is usually perfectly straightforward. The only difficulty might be in locating the obturator foramen, which has to be done by guesswork. However, the tip of the tunneller can usually be felt against the membrane after successive passes with it from below have been made. The only other problem that is sometimes seen is an extension of infection and frank pus along the graft into the iliac wound. If this is present then extensive irrigation using a weak antiseptic solution should take place once the graft has been exposed. This is usually sufficient to deal with the problem as, once the old graft has been removed, there should be no further difficulty. As new graft material is being stitched end to end with existing graft material, infection does not usually persist or cause a problem. If there is any doubt about distal run-off below the femoral artery, then on-table arteriography should be performed before the procedure is undertaken. If this shows a relatively poor run-off then the operation may fail.

POSTOPERATIVE CARE

Antibiotics should continue for a full course of treatment and a careful watch kept on the new wounds to detect infection early. The groin wound usually heals by first intention, but occasionally it has to be allowed to granulate.

RESULTS

The results are usually good,[1,2] provided that reasonable distal vessels are available. If the run-off is poor, it is probably best to use a vein graft rather than Dacron or PTFE.

OTHER ROUTES

If the procedure described here is not feasible, an alternative solution is to take a graft from the opposite iliac artery across the pelvis passing behind the abdominal muscles and then subcutaneously along the medial side of the leg to the popliteal artery in order to avoid the infected area. Another very rarely used route is via the gluteal foramen deep inside the pelvis with the graft passing into the leg posteriorly. It is usually unnecessary to use either of these routes.

REFERENCES

1   Van Det R J, Brands L C 1981 The obturator foramen bypass: an alternative procedure in iliofemoral artery revascularisation. Surgery 89: 543–547
2   Geroulakis G, Parvin S D, Bell P R F 1988 Obturator foramen bypass: the alternative route for sepsis in the femoral triangle. Acta Chirurgica Scandinavica 154: 111–112

Chapter 8

Popliteal aneurysm

Introduction

Popliteal aneurysms are relatively uncommon (Fig. 8.1), but getting more common as the population ages. They are frequently bilateral and often associated with an abdominal aortic aneurysm.[1] They rarely rupture but present with acute ischaemia due to distal embolisation or sudden thrombosis, when surgery becomes necessary, often as an emergency.

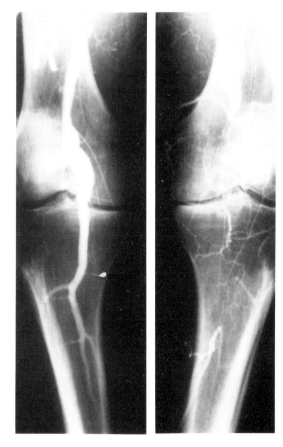

Fig. 8.1

Angiogram of popliteal aneurysm—still patent on the right, but occluded on the left.

INDICATIONS FOR SURGERY

With acute ischaemia, surgical treatment is mandatory but fibrinolysis, with streptokinase,[2] urokinase or tissue plasminogen activator given directly into the artery, may be needed first (Fig. 8.2). If an aneurysm is found incidentally, there is some controversy about treatment. Some surgeons believe that these lesions should be watched and dealt with only if they give rise to symptoms, while others favour a more aggressive approach to treatment. The results of surgery are so good[3] and the consequences of thrombosis or embolisation potentially so serious[4] (almost inevitable limb loss) that an operation should usually be done to replace a palpable lesion confirmed by ultrasound.

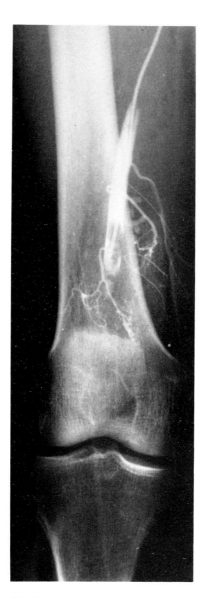

Fig. 8.2
Catheter in the femoral artery above an area of thrombosis—low-dose streptokinase is being injected directly into the thrombus.

THE OPERATION

As for the aorta, the aneurysm sac does not need to be removed and, because the vessels are often larger than normal above and below the sac, artificial graft materials such as Dacron or PTFE can be used successfully. The best graft is, however, vein[3] and the long or short saphenous vein is usually available. The latter in particular, because of its location, should be considered if the posterior approach is being used. If this is not available, however, then the long saphenous vein should be used. The results of surgery are excellent, as there is usually a reasonable run-off into the foot, unless thrombosis or embolism have occurred. Two approaches are possible, the medial or the posterior.

Medial approach

This approach is the simplest and has the advantage that it avoids vital structures in the popliteal fossa while allowing access to the long saphenous vein. The disadvantage is that the sac is not decompressed and may act as an obstruction to the graft; however, it should be the operation of choice.

Procedure

The patient is placed in the supine position and the extent of the lesion will easily be felt. A medial incision must first be made, as for exposure of the popliteal artery above the knee (Fig. 8.3). The artery will be larger than normal and should be controlled by a sling just above the aneurysm (Fig. 8.4). A second incision should be made below the knee, as for exposure of the infrageniculate popliteal artery (p. 130), and a sling placed around the popliteal artery below the aneurysm (Fig. 8.5). A run-off vessel can usually be identified on the preoperative angiogram and found in this position. The aneurysm must then be isolated by ligatures tied above and below the sac (Fig. 8.6) after the patient has been heparinised. Two approaches can now be taken, but a graft placed end-to-side above and below the sac is the simplest and least dangerous method of bypassing the lesion. The long saphenous vein, if it is available, should be removed, as described on page 116, using the upper larger portion if possible. It should be reversed and passed through a tunnel made between the popliteal artery above and below the aneurysm, taking care not to damage the sac or kink the

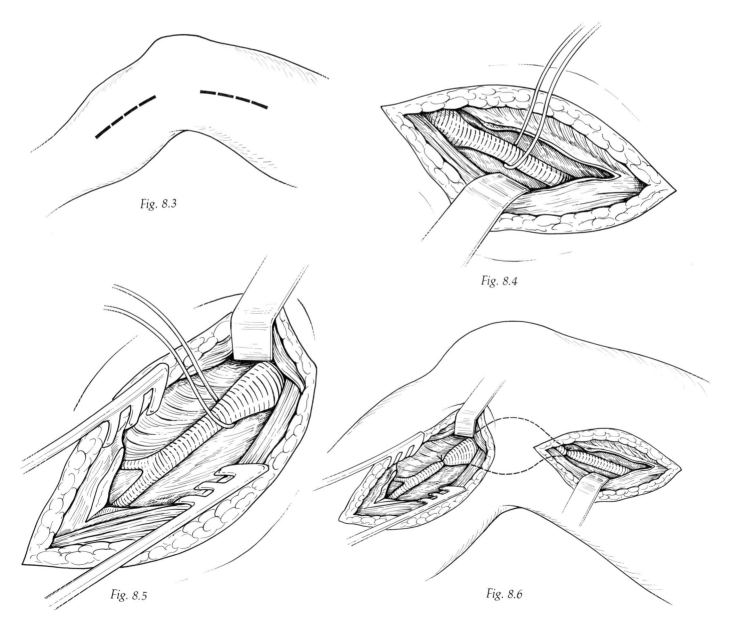

Fig. 8.3

Fig. 8.4

Fig. 8.5

Fig. 8.6

vein in any way. The lower anastomosis is first constructed as described on page 133 and the leg then straightened. The upper anastomosis is then completed in the same way, thereby by-passing the lesion (Fig. 8.7).

Alternatively, but only rarely, the sac can be tied and the vessels divided, clamps having first been placed on the vessels prior to division. The sac should not be unduly disturbed until distal control is obtained otherwise distal emboli can occur. A tunnel should then be made between the two incisions taking care again not to place the tunnelling forceps through the sac as difficult bleeding will occur. Because the sac offers obstruction to a graft, this technique is suitable only for smaller aneurysms. Having done this and assessed the size of the artery above and below, either externally supported PTFE, Dacron, or preferably a piece of long saphenous vein, is used to bridge the gap (Fig. 8.8). The graft is then tunnelled between the two wounds and sutured end-to-end (Fig. 8.9).

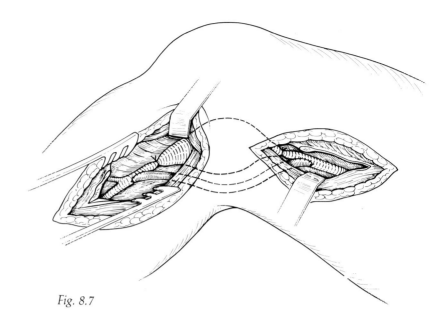

Fig. 8.7

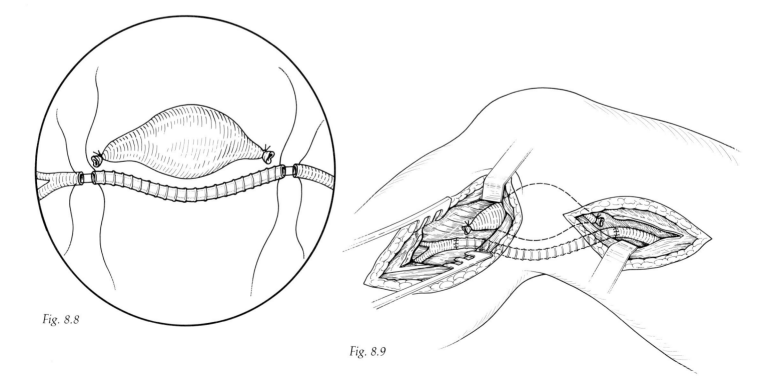

Fig. 8.8

Fig. 8.9

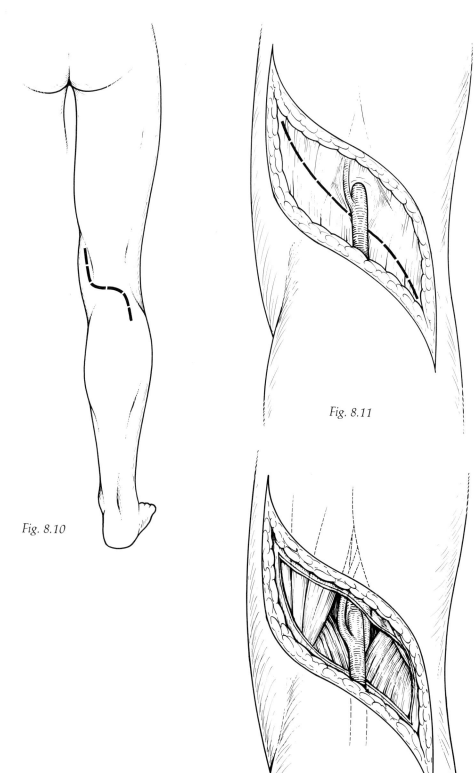

Fig. 8.10

Fig. 8.11

Fig. 8.12

Posterior approach

This approach should always be used if the sac is large and liable to cause obstruction to a medially placed graft. Before placing the patient, a decision about which graft is to be used should be taken. If the proximal long saphenous vein is to be used, this should be harvested first (see p. 116), the wound closed and the patient then placed face down. Sometimes a piece of long saphenous vein can be obtained from the medial side of the leg with the patient in the face-down position; alternatively, the short saphenous vein can be used. The popliteal fossa is exposed through an S-shaped incision (Fig. 8.10), or alternatively, a vertical incision can be used. After cutting through the skin, the short saphenous vein will be seen crossing the space and should be preserved in case it can be used as a graft later (Fig. 8.11). The deep fascia is incised (Fig. 8.12) exposing the popliteal contents. The short saphenous vein can either be removed and used as a graft, ligated and divided, or retracted to one side.

Dissection of the skin flaps will expose the aneurysm and the popliteal vein and nerves which are usually adherent to it (Fig. 8.13). The gastrocnemius muscle should be divided as necessary proximally, the semi-tendinosus medially and the biceps femoris (laterally) should be separated to allow access to the neck of the sac. This is usually prior to the dis-appearance of the artery through the adductor magnus. Great care should be taken at this stage as the popliteal vein is usually stretched over the sac along with the medial popliteal nerve, but these structures can easily be seen and avoided. Attempts should not be made to look for branches of the sac as this

will lead to unnecessary dissection and possibly damage the nerves mentioned previously. The sac should be handled carefully until distal control is achieved, otherwise emboli can be dislodged. Once control of the proximal and distal artery has been achieved by careful dis-section, the sac should be opened longitudinally (Fig. 8.14), thrombus removed and any branches that are visible oversewn in the same way as one would oversew the branches of the abdominal aorta when dealing with an aneurysm (Fig. 8.15). Once this has been done, the artery above and below the sac is divided (Fig. 8.16) and the graft inserted. If dividing the posterior wall proves to be a problem, this can be left

intact and the graft inlayed as for an aortic aneurysm. Again, depending on the size of the vessels, Dacron, PTFE or vein can be used. Because of the patient's position, the short saphenous vein offers the best conduit, but if this is not available and saphenous vein is required, a separate incision along the medial side of the leg will allow access to the lower part of the long saphenous vein. Alternatively, a piece of vein is taken from the groin as already described. Once the procedure is finished, the space is drained and the sac sutured over the artery (Fig. 8.17). Alternatively, if the sac is large and causing obstruction most of it can be excised.

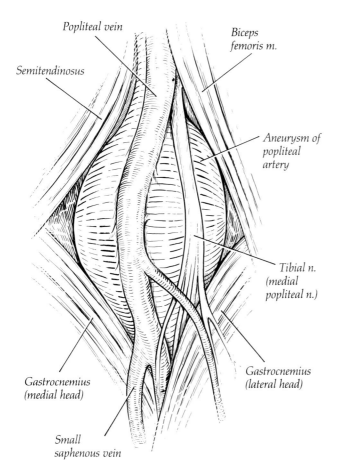

Fig. 8.13

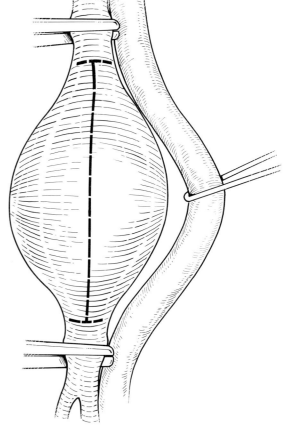

Fig. 8.14

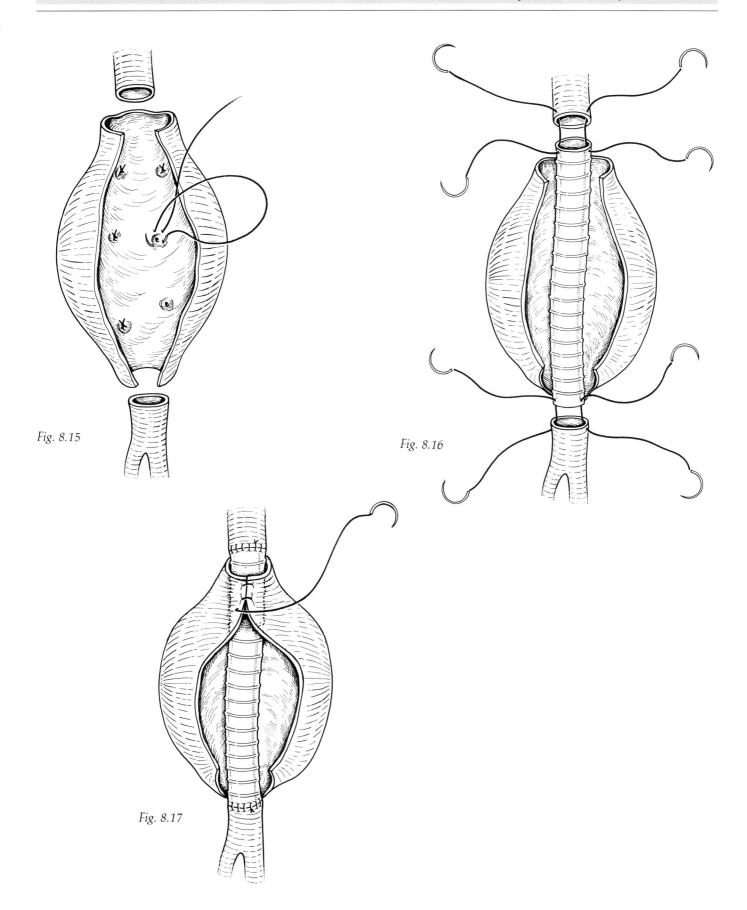

Fig. 8.15

Fig. 8.16

Fig. 8.17

ASSESSMENT OF THE PROCEDURE

The foot should be inspected after completion of the anastomosis and its preoperative insertion into a sterile transparent plastic bag will facilitate this. It is also wise to do a completion arteriogram, as described on page 16. Failure to see the run-off vessels beyond the graft is an indication for exploration and the passage of a Fogarty catheter, as described on page 17.

PROBLEMS WITH THE OPERATION

Provided proper planning is done prior to starting, there should be no difficulties. The main problem of the medial approach is that, if it is attempted with too large an aneurysmal sac, there is insufficient space for the graft to pass. With the posterior approach great care must be taken to avoid damage to the medial popliteal nerve and the popliteal vein. If the sac is incised medially, with the vein and nerve dissected laterally, there should be no difficulty. It is important to obtain an arteriogram before starting the operation to ensure that the distal run-off is available and also to locate where the distal graft should go. If the run-off is into a single tibial vessel, then the vein should always be used. The sac should not be handled unduly until the distal vessel is properly controlled, otherwise distal irretrievable embolisation leading to trash foot can occur. A decision about which graft to use should be taken before placing the patient in the face-down position. Vein is the best graft and, if the popliteal artery above and below the aneurysm is large, then the widest part of the long saphenous vein will be needed. This is, of course, the proximal part which should be removed first from groin to above the knee. This wound is then closed and the patient turned over to allow a posterior approach. If vein is not available, or if an artificial graft is being used, it should probably be one of the newer externally supported types which do not kink when the knee is bent. If the leg is acutely ischaemic with a poor run-off, then grafting will be unsuccessful under these circumstances: fibrinolysis as an alternative should be considered prior to undertaking surgical correction of the lesion.[2]

POSTOPERATIVE CARE

Bleeding should, of course, be looked for and the circulation of the foot examined regularly. If an artificial graft has been used, then postoperative long-term antiplatelet drugs or anticoagulant therapy should be considered. The other leg should always be examined as these aneurysms are frequently bilateral. Once the patient has recovered, the other side should be dealt with electively, usually within 6 months.

RESULTS

The results of this operation are usually excellent, with long-term patency in excess of 90% for those procedures undertaken electively using vein. Emergency operations required because of distal embolisation have a much poorer prognosis with a high amputation rate.

REFERENCES

1 Guvendik L, Bloor K, Charlesworth D 1980 Popliteal aneurysm: sinister harbinger of sudden catastrophe. British Journal of Surgery 67: 294–296
2 Porter J M, Taylor I M 1985 Current status of thrombolytic therapy. Journal of Vascular Surgery 2: 239–249
3 Anton G E, Hertzer N R, Beven E G, O'Hara P J, Krajewski L P 1986 Surgical management of popliteal aneurysms. Trends in presentation, treatment and results from 1952–1984. Journal of Vascular Surgery 3: 125–129
4 Whitehouse W M, Wakefield T W, Graham L M et al 1983 Limb-threatening potential of arteriosclerotic popliteal artery aneurysm. Surgery 93: 694–698

Chapter 9

Popliteal artery entrapment syndrome and cystic adventitial disease

Introduction

These two conditions are relatively rare, but they can cause severe claudication and occasionally critical ischaemia in young adults. Because they are rare, an eminently treatable lesion will be missed unless the condition is considered.

POPLITEAL ARTERY ENTRAPMENT SYNDROME

The popliteal artery normally passes down the middle of the popliteal fossa, the vessel would then normally pass down the leg between the two heads of the gastrocnemius muscle. Anomalies in the insertion of the medial head of gastrocnemius, or passage of the artery through the muscle itself, can lead to its entrapment.

Presentation

As mentioned previously, the lesion occurs in young adults with claudication or severe ischaemia.[1] Symptoms frequently arise after prolonged exercise and the vessel can thrombose or be prone to aneurysmal dilatation beyond the area of compression. There is some disagreement about classification, but from a practical point of view there are two main lesions. In the first, the artery is placed medially passing around a normally inserted gastrocnemius muscle (Fig. 9.1) and in the second type the medial head of gastrocnemius arises more laterally than normal, compressing the artery (Fig. 9.2). There are various subtypes in the relationship to the muscle causing compression of the artery.[2]

Distal examination might be entirely normal unless the possibility of entrapment is borne in mind. The important physical sign to remember is that the pulse will disappear if the patient plantarflexes against resistance. Arteriography will show a classical picture of deviation of the popliteal artery with a cut-off in flow on plantarflexion of the foot.

Treatment

All cases should be operated upon as the condition will otherwise lead to thrombosis and acute ischaemia.

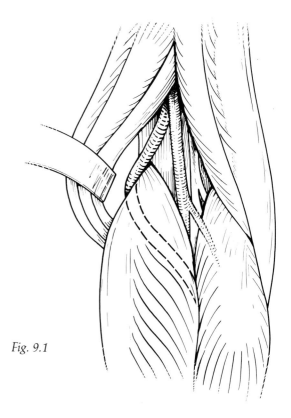

Fig. 9.1

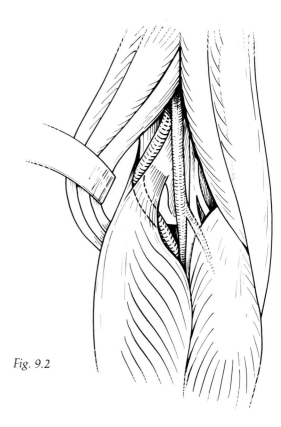

Fig. 9.2

Procedure

The patient should be placed in the prone position and a posterior approach used. A medial approach to bypass the area completely, as for popliteal aneurysm, is possible, but the lesion is best examined directly through a posterior incision. The incision is made as for a popliteal aneurysm and the vessel approached in a similar way (see p. 93). The heads of the gastrocnemius muscles will be seen and the contents of the popliteal fossa will differ from normal in that the artery will clearly be displaced medially. If, on arteriography, the artery appears to be normal, then it can be treated by division of the aberrant muscle and relocation of the artery to its normal position. This is difficult, however, because the vessel is frequently bound tightly to the back of the knee joint with fibrous tissue. If it proves impossible to free it, then it should be divided above and below the area of entrapment and the ends of the trapped artery ligated (Fig. 9.3). The popliteal artery can then be re-constituted by a vein graft (Fig. 9.4) taken either from the short saphenous vein or, prior to the procedure, from the upper part of the long saphenous vein in the groin, as for popliteal aneurysm (p. 95). The results of this type of approach are excellent and will return the patient to normal.

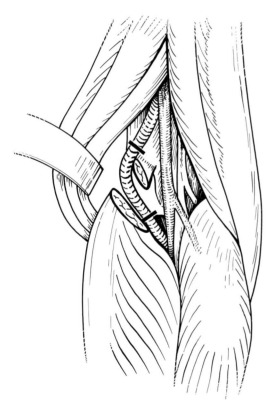

Fig. 9.3

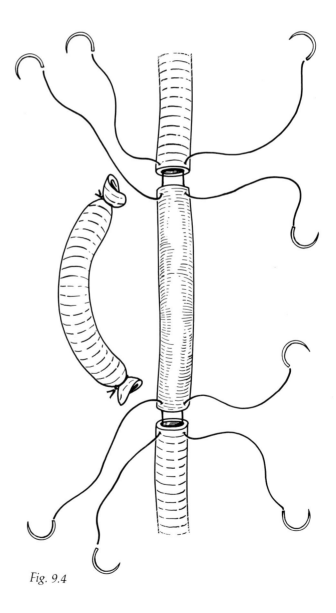

Fig. 9.4

CYSTIC DEGENERATION OF THE POPLITEAL ARTERY

This condition again affects adults and can be confused with entrapment. The cause is unknown but one of many theories attributes the condition to the inclusion of mucin-secreting cells within the adventitia during development.[3] These cells secrete a mucinous material and produce a large cyst, or multiple cysts, which encroach upon the arterial lumen, causing eventual occlusion with ischaemia and thrombosis.

Presentation
In contrast to entrapment, this condition affects older men—usually middle aged—and appears very suddenly, although a history of claudication is possible. On examination, the pulses are usually absent and the cystic lesion cannot usually be felt. Arteriographic findings are classical, the tapering artery produces what is known as a scimitar sign. The diagnosis is usually confirmed by CAT scanning or ultrasound, which show the lesion in the arterial wall.

Treatment
It is possible, using ultrasound or CAT scan control, to aspirate the cyst from time to time thereby relieving the condition. A better alternative is to explore the lesion using a posterior approach, incise the cyst with a scalpel (Fig. 9.5) and remove the edges of the sac, which will solve the problem. If the arteries thrombose, or the cyst is large, then an alternative is simply to mobilise the artery as for a popliteal aneurysm, ligate it above and below the cystic area and bypass the lesion with a graft of either the short or long saphenous vein (Fig. 9.6), using an end-to-end anastomosis, as described on page 28. The medial approach can be used, bypassing the lesion with a vein graft sutured to the popliteal artery above and below the cystic area, but the posterior approach is probably to be preferred in order to make the diagnosis accurately.

Results of treatment
These are excellent if the cyst is bypassed with a vein graft; aspirations or incision of the lesion can lead to a recurrence.

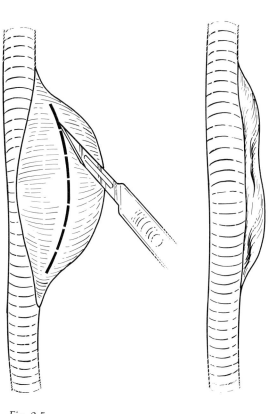

Fig. 9.5

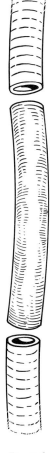

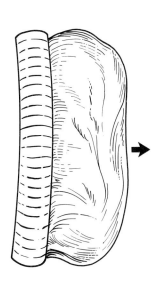

Fig. 9.6

REFERENCES

1   Hallett J W Jr, Greenwood L H, Robinson J G 1985 Lower extremity
      arterial disease in young adults. A systematic approach to early
      diagnosis. Annals of Surgery 202: 647–652
2   Delaney T A, Gonzalez L L 1971 Occlusion of the popliteal artery due
      to muscular entrapment. Surgery 69: 97–99
3   Haid S P, Conn J Jr, Bergan J J 1970 Cystic adventitial disease of the
      popliteal artery. Archives of Surgery 101: 765–768

Chapter 10

Femoropopliteal occlusion

Introduction

The popliteal artery is usually occluded in the region of the adductor canal with a run-off vessel above (Fig. 10.1) or below the knee (Fig. 10.2). Sometimes an isolated patent segment of this vessel can also be seen (Fig. 10.3). The approaches to occlusions above and below the knee are different and will be described separately. When the vessels are blocked lower down the leg, operations to the crural vessels are described as femorodistal or femorocrural.

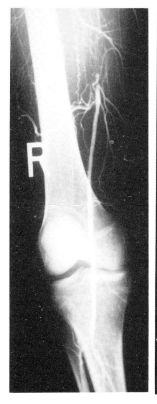

Fig. 10.1
Femoropopliteal occlusion with patent run-off vessel above the knee.

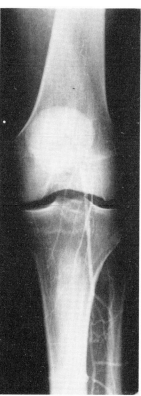

Fig. 10.2
Femoropopliteal occlusion with patent run-off vessel below the knee.

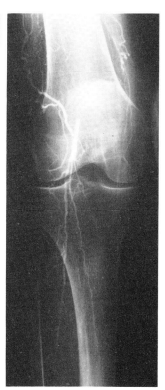

Fig. 10.3
Isolated patent segment of popliteal artery.

FEMOROPOPLITEAL ABOVE-KNEE GRAFT

This procedure has been a classical operation in vascular surgery for many years. Charles Rob[1] popularised the operation using the patient's own long saphenous vein, reversed to bypass an obstruction usually in the adductor canal. Although the long saphenous vein gives the best results,[2] a number of graft substitutes have been produced which give acceptable results in this position. If there is any doubt about the adequacy of the run-off, then an operation above the knee should not be performed; the graft should be taken to the popliteal artery below the knee.

INDICATIONS FOR THIS OPERATION

Indications, as always in vascular surgery, would be for severe claudication or critical ischaemia. If rest pain is present, an obstruction at this level is usually accompanied by other obstructions distally or proximally. The indications for operating on a patient with claudication will vary with the surgeon and the patient, but as a general rule patients should not have surgery for claudication unless they are significantly affected by the symptoms. Although the results are relatively good, there are possible complications which could at worst result in limb loss. The improvement gained from stopping smoking and exercising[3] should be maximal before surgery is undertaken and the possibility of angioplasty fully explored.

PREOPERATIVE PROCEDURES

A good preoperative arteriogram is important and both proximal and distal run-off to the ankle must adequately be seen. Because infection in vascular procedures, particularly where artificial grafts are used, is a potential disaster, the patient should be given a prophylactic antibiotic either as a single dose or for 24 hours commencing with the premedication. The appropriate drugs are discussed in Chapter 1. Skin preparation, both in the ward and operating theatre, should extend from the mid-abdomen to the foot.

If there is any doubt about the adequacy of inflow into the limb, suggested either by a weak femoral pulse or a suspicious X-ray of the aortoiliac region, an inflow study of some kind should be performed. There are very few adequate tests to assess inflow. However, the best one is probably the papaverine test, even though it is invasive. This test has already been described in detail in Chapter 1. Briefly, after hyperaemia caused by intra-arterial papaverine, a drop in pressure of 20% distal to the narrowed segment suggests a proximal lesion.[4,5]

The test can also be performed at the time of arteriography using a catheter on which are mounted two miniature transducers which can detect a pressure drop across the stenosis (see Ch. 1). An advantage of this is that, should a significant stenosis be discovered, angioplasty can be performed at that time and the result of dilatation assessed by final pressure measurements.

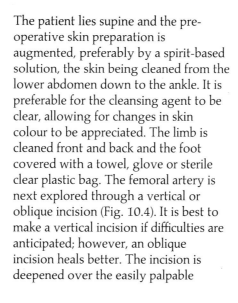

Fig. 10.4

OPERATIVE DETAILS

The patient lies supine and the pre-operative skin preparation is augmented, preferably by a spirit-based solution, the skin being cleaned from the lower abdomen down to the ankle. It is preferable for the cleansing agent to be clear, allowing for changes in skin colour to be appreciated. The limb is cleaned front and back and the foot covered with a towel, glove or sterile clear plastic bag. The femoral artery is next explored through a vertical or oblique incision (Fig. 10.4). It is best to make a vertical incision if difficulties are anticipated; however, an oblique incision heals better. The incision is deepened over the easily palpable femoral pulse dividing the deep fascia (Fig. 10.5) and the small vessels which cross the area transversely—these are, of course, ligated. The deep fascia over the femoral artery and vein is then cut longitudinally using a pair of curved scissors. The artery with the vein lying medially will now be apparent. Provided the patient has a good inflow with a palpable femoral pulse, finding the artery will not be a problem. Make sure that the incision in the fascia is not made too medially as the saphenous vein may be damaged and lymphatics can be cut. By picking up the fascia close to the artery and using a pair of blunt scissors on each side of the vessel, further dissection will then be possible (Fig. 10.6).

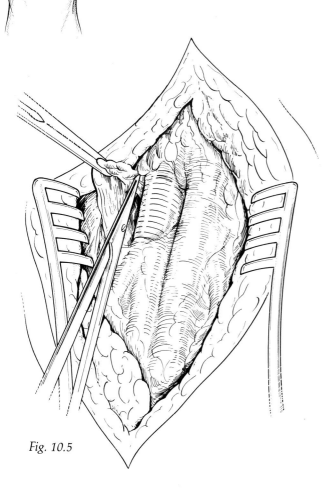

Fig. 10.5

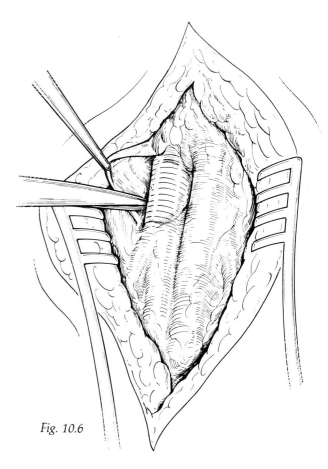

Fig. 10.6

Using a pair of right-angled forceps and a gentle opening and closing movement, it should be possible to pass them behind the artery (Fig. 10.7). A silastic sling is then grasped by the forceps and pulled around the vessel, in this way control of the common femoral artery is achieved. Gentle traction on the sling will now allow sharp dissection with curved scissors to proceed up the common femoral and down the superficial femoral arteries. The site of the profunda femoris will be seen as the point where the femoral artery becomes slightly narrower—this is where the bifurcation can be found. A sling is now placed in a similar fashion around the superficial femoral artery (Fig. 10.8). By gentle traction on the two slings already placed, the origin of the profunda femoris will be seen. Careful attention must be paid to the origin of this vessel in case there is a posterior or medial branch which has to be separately controlled. Once the profunda origin has been isolated a silastic sling is placed around it (Fig. 10.9). Sharp dissection along the artery will now expose a small vein crossing the profunda. This has to be ligated and divided. Once this has been done the two major branches of the profunda femoris artery will be seen.

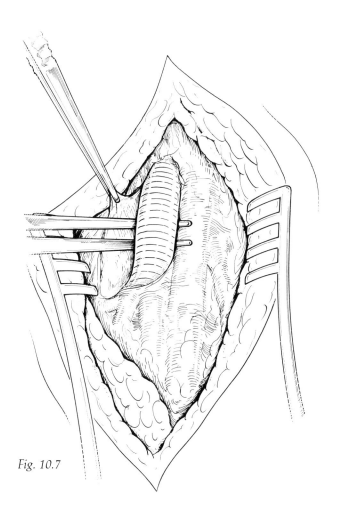

Fig. 10.7

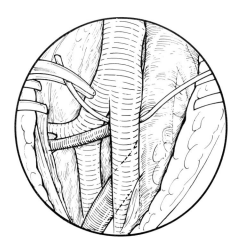

Fig. 10.8

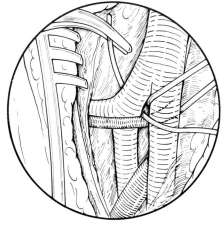

Fig. 10.9

Using careful dissection as previously mentioned the two branches can now be isolated and slings placed separately around each (Figs 10.10 and 10.11). If any further access to the profunda is required, the profunda femoris vein which crosses this vessel lower down may need to be divided as for profundaplasty. At this stage, slings should be around the superficial femoral, common femoral and branches of the profunda femoris artery (Fig. 10.12), and all other slings can be removed.

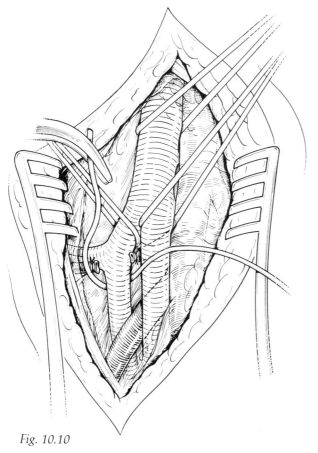

Fig. 10.10

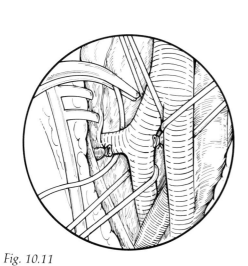

Fig. 10.11

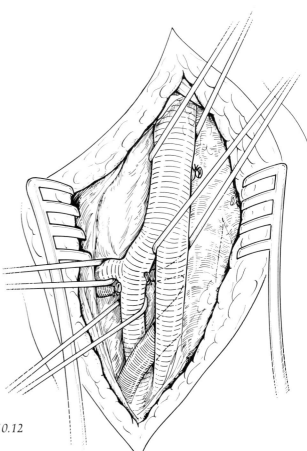

Fig. 10.12

Having completed the groin dissection, the femoral artery above the knee is next exposed. An incision is made along the anterior border of the sartorius muscle (Fig. 10.13), taking care to avoid the long saphenous vein. The deep fascia is divided longitudinally, looking carefully for the long saphenous nerve which perforates the fascia near this point and becomes superficial (Fig. 10.14). Division of this nerve results in a great deal of morbidity postoperatively and must be avoided at all costs. Division of the fascia behind the nerve will expose the sartorius muscle (Fig. 10.15), which is displaced backwards (Fig. 10.16), and fibrofatty tissue is then encountered.

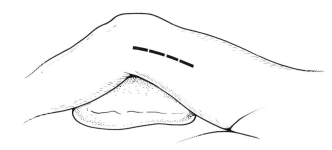

Fig. 10.13

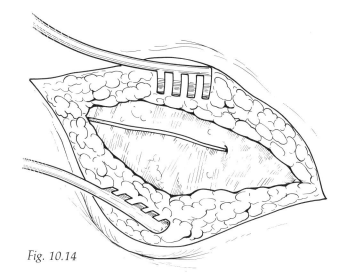

Fig. 10.14

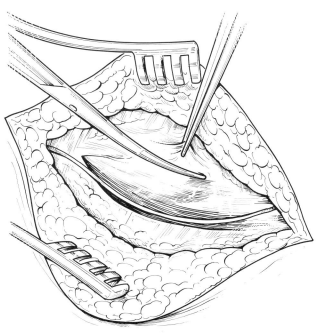

Fig. 10.15

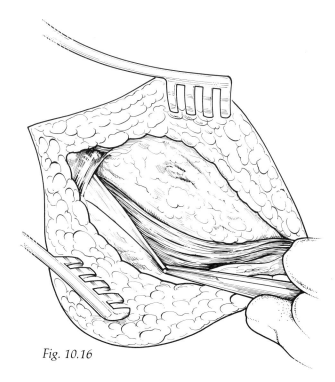

Fig. 10.16

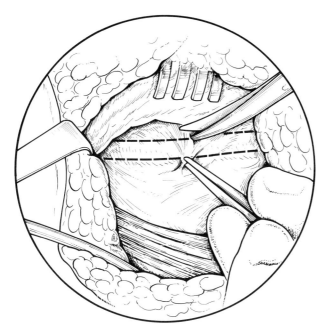

Fig. 10.17

Using a pair of forceps, this tissue is grasped and divided with scissors (Fig. 10.17). As this dissection proceeds, a finger can now be introduced into this tissue and palpation behind the femur will reveal the femoral artery close to the bone. The knee should be flexed during this dissection and the leg slightly externally rotated. Once the artery is palpated the fascia over it is grasped by forceps and divided. A right-angled clamp is then placed around the artery and a silastic sling passed (Fig. 10.18). Two slings are passed in this way and a segment of artery is then available, gentle traction on the slings will allow as much length as necessary to be exposed (Fig. 10.19) (usually 5–7 cm). Any branches should be controlled and protected.

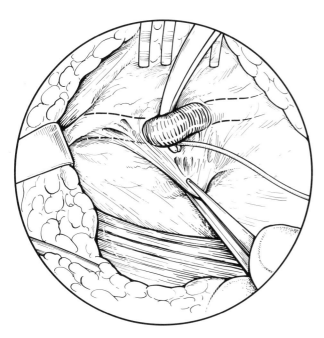

Fig. 10.18

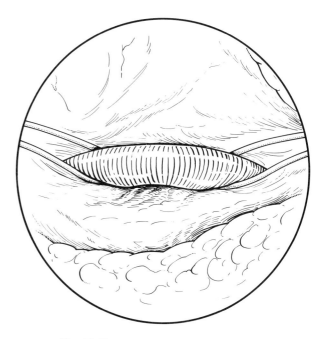

Fig. 10.19

A decision must now be made about which graft is to be used. The alternatives available will be either the long saphenous vein, a segment of artificial material such as PTFE, Dacron or umbilical vein graft or vein from the arm. A decision about which material to use is often a personal one, but there is no doubt that results from the use of long saphenous vein are best; however, this has to be set against the possible usefulness of the long saphenous vein if this is required later for an anastomosis below the knee. Artificial grafts, generally speaking, can produce equivalent results when inserted above the knee.[6] For this reason it might be prudent to use one and save the vein for later.

Removal of the long saphenous vein
This can either be used in situ or can be removed and reversed, which is the classical procedure. The in situ technique is described later for procedures below the knee and reference should be made to that operation if it is intended to use the vein in this way. However, recent publications suggest that the same results can be obtained from reversed or in situ vein grafts in this location.[7] After exposure of the femoral and popliteal vessels, the saphenous vein should be removed either through a continuous incision, or through multiple vertical incisions with skin bridges between them (Fig. 10.20). This approach is associated with better healing. However,

provided that the skin edges are not undermined, a continuous incision is easier to use and heals as well as the shorter ones; undermining can be avoided by preoperative duplex scanning of the vein.[8] The vein is first of all seen at the top of the leg, where it should be visible in the groin incision (Fig. 10.21). The saphenofemoral junction is defined and the vein divided flush (Fig. 10.22) with the femoral and followed downwards, dividing the skin as the dissection proceeds in order to make the incision over the vein rather than away from it, thereby avoiding undermining of the skin flap.

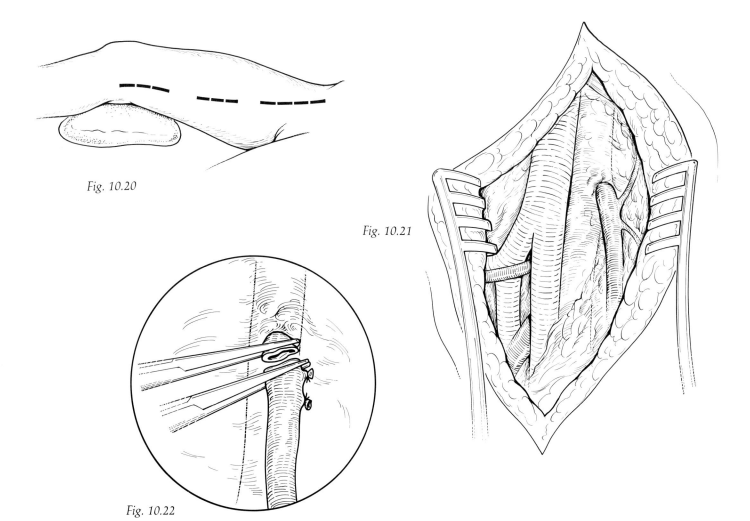

Fig. 10.20

Fig. 10.21

Fig. 10.22

Skin bridges (if a continuous incision is to be avoided) are maintained as in Figure 10.23. The distal end of the vein is divided (Fig. 10.24).

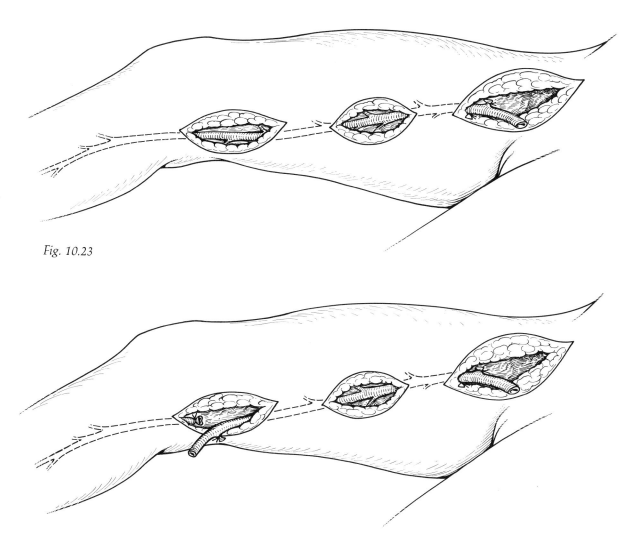

Fig. 10.23

Fig. 10.24

As the dissection proceeds, the branches of the vein are identified and doubly ligated, those branches behind the skin bridges being divided after appropriate retraction. The upper end is pulled towards the middle incision (Fig. 10.25), which puts the remaining branches on tension, facilitating their division (Fig. 10.26). The adequacy of the ligatures on the branches is tested by reversing the vein and gently injecting heparinised saline down it. The temptation to do this under high pressure in order to distend the vein should be resisted as damage will otherwise occur.

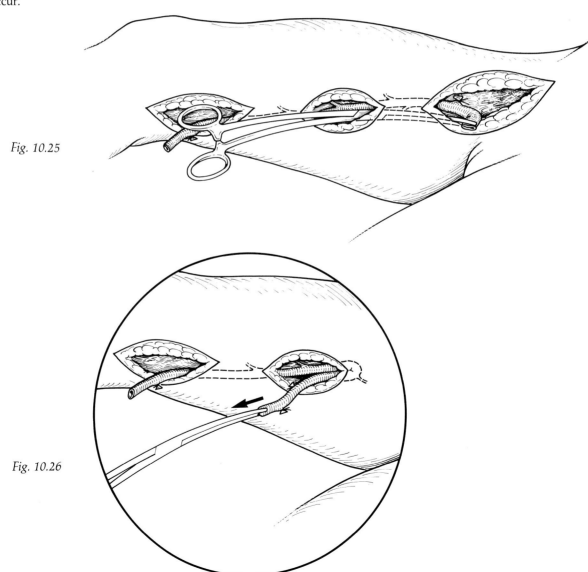

Fig. 10.25

Fig. 10.26

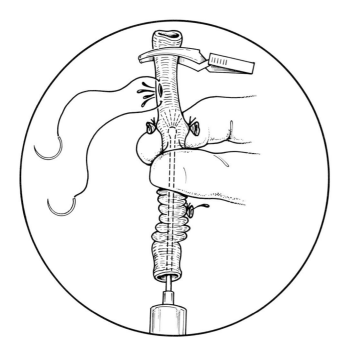

Fig. 10.27

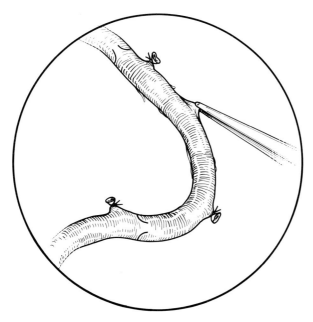

Fig 10.28

Any defects are sutured (Fig. 10.27) with 60 monofilament stitches. Once this has been done, gentle distension will allow any pieces of adventitia causing narrowing to be stripped off (Fig. 10.28).

Using Dacron

Generally speaking, Dacron does not give very good results when used in this position, although some authors have suggested that good results[9] can be obtained. If it is used, then 8 mm diameter woven or knitted material is acceptable. The exact length of graft required should be estimated after the material has been passed through a tunnel between the two incisions. This will be described later.

PTFE

This material does not stretch—the main point to remember about it is that the opening in the artery must be precisely equivalent to the diameter of the graft otherwise tearing of one or other will occur. The material slips very easily through a tunnel and a 6 mm graft can be used.

Externally supported grafts

Both Dacron and PTFE can now be obtained with an external support which prevents kinking. These grafts are best used when the knee joint is crossed, although definite evidence of their superiority in this situation is still lacking.

Umbilical vein

This material is very friable and has to be placed accurately through a tunneller before any anastomosis is performed: it cannot be moved later. In general, the net does not need to be incorporated into the anastomosis but can be tacked down with a few sutures once the anastomosis has been completed.

INSERTION OF GRAFT AND THE ANASTOMOSIS

It is usually best to perform the distal anastomosis first, but either can be done depending on the preference of the operator. The popliteal artery above the knee is occluded with vascular clamps, using minimal pressure to occlude the vessel. Before this is done, if adequate arteriography has not been obtained preoperatively, then an on-table angiogram should be performed now, as described on page 28. Using a scalpel with no. 11 blade, a vertical incision is made at the chosen point of the artery about 2 cm in length (Fig. 10.29). The final dimensions of the arteriotomy can be completed with right-angled scissors (Fig. 10.30), the clamp is released distally to ensure that adequate back bleeding occurs (Fig. 10.31).

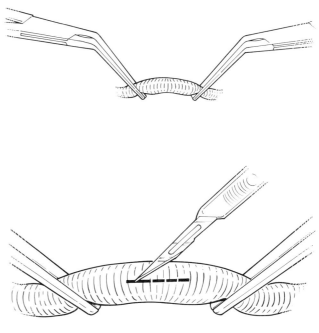

Fig. 10.29

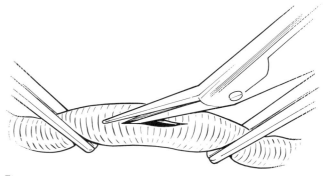

Fig. 10.30

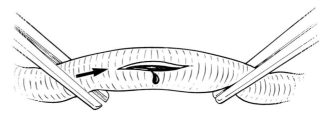

Fig. 10.31

A tunneller is now passed up the leg from below, or down from above—the latter is usually easier. The tunneller is a curved metal tube with a central obturator to prevent trauma to tissue. If it is introduced above (the best route) it should be passed along the course of the superficial femoral artery, passing gradually deeper as the leg is traversed. Just above the adductor canal it is passed backwards into the posterior compartment to emerge next to the popliteal vessels. A finger inserted at the lower opening will serve to guide the tunneller (Fig. 10.32). The obturator is removed and a pair of forceps are passed down the tunneller to grasp the graft which is then pulled through (Fig. 10.33). The tunneller is then removed by pulling it out of the wound in a downwards direction making sure that the graft is not also pulled out in the process. If a tunneller is not available a similar tunnel can be made with two long forceps passed upwards and downwards until they meet.

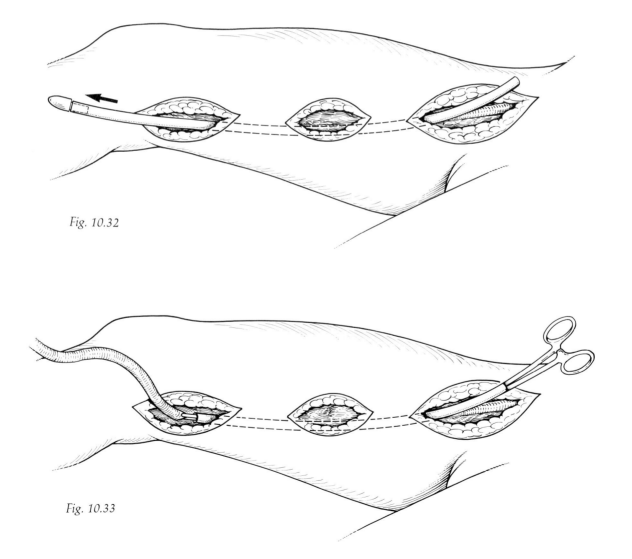

Fig. 10.32

Fig. 10.33

The graft is next cut obliquely to fit the arteriotomy and the corners trimmed (Fig. 10.34). At this stage it is best to inject heparinised saline down the graft to ensure that it is not kinked in its tunnel. If the saphenous vein has been used it should, of course, be reversed before being passed through the tunneller. There are several ways of doing this anastomosis, as described in Chapter 5, and they will be described briefly here. Monofilament vascular sutures such as Prolene are next inserted into the heel of the graft, which is first sutured to the proximal end of the arteriotomy ensuring that the stitch is tied on the outside of the vessel (Fig. 10.35) and then passed over and over along one side of the anastomosis reaching almost to the toe. The other end of the stitch is then passed behind the graft and used to complete the anastomosis along the other side (Figs 10.36 and 10.37); this again stops short of the apex of the graft. The toe is then completed by inserting four or five interrupted sutures, which are tied after they have all been inserted (Fig. 10.38). If the vessel is large, which is usually the case, the anastomosis can be completed with continuous sutures, one of the sutures in Figure 10.36 being taken around the back of the vessel (Fig. 10.37). Alternatively the anastomosis can be performed by using two separate sutures at the heel and toe (Fig. 10.39).

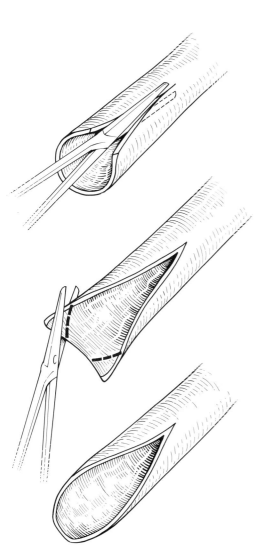

Fig. 10.34

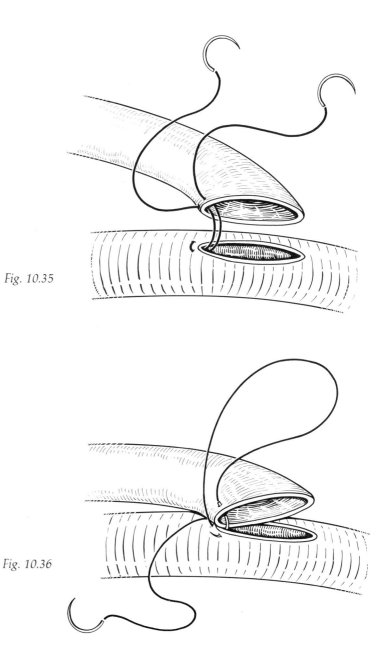

Fig. 10.35

Fig. 10.36

One side is completed and tied and the remaining needle used to complete the other side ensuring that the stitch finishes in the middle so as to avoid blind sutures in corners (Fig. 10.40). If the posterior wall is inaccessible, a third technique is to suture the vein from the inside using an over-and-over technique so that a loop of suture is always on the inside of the vessel. Whichever method is used, before the last stitch is inserted, the distal clamp must be released to ensure that there is adequate back bleeding.

Once this anastomosis has been completed the graft can be clamped just above the suture line. The patient will have been heparinised prior to clamping the vessels. Attention is now turned to the upper end—clamps are placed across the common femoral artery, profunda and superficial femoral. The graft is put on tension—in the case of a human umbilical vein graft this will already have been done as the graft will otherwise not pull through the tissue. The leg is straightened and an arteriotomy is made in the common femoral artery passing across the mouth of the profunda femoris. If the profunda is in reasonable condition, the arteriotomy can be made in the common femoral artery. This is often the case and it is easier to sew the graft to it.

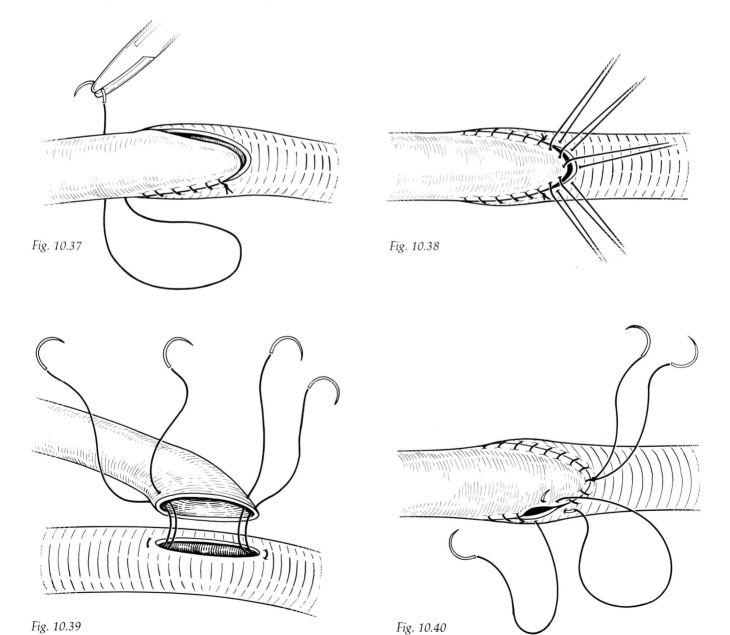

Fig. 10.37

Fig. 10.38

Fig. 10.39

Fig. 10.40

The vein is cut obliquely so that its orifice matches the femoral arteriotomy (Fig. 10.41). The anastomosis is now fashioned in one of the three ways already described for the lower anastomosis (Figs 10.42 and 10.43). Before the suture is tied, the proximal and distal clamps must be released to ensure that back bleeding is adequate and that proximal flow is also sufficient to displace any clot in the vessel. Once the clamps are released, bleeding is looked for at both anastomoses and any obvious haemorrhage stopped with extra sutures. If simple oozing occurs, this can usually be controlled with pressure or by applying some form of haemostatic gauze.

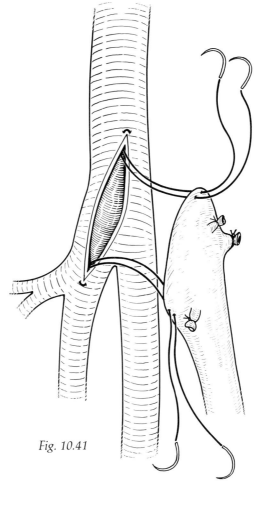

Fig. 10.41

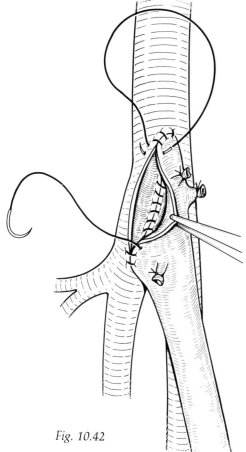

Fig. 10.42

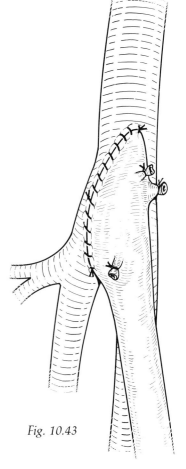

Fig. 10.43

ASSESSMENT OF THE PROCEDURE

Even though the pulse in the graft both proximal to and beyond the anastomosis appears to be adequate, it is essential that the operation is assessed. The popular techniques are on-table arteriography, measurement of flow, measurement of pressure proximal to and distal to the anastomosis, or the use of a Doppler probe to assess forward flow. If a Doppler probe is available, then a demonstration of forward flow is probably sufficient. If an electromagnetic flow meter is available, this can be placed around the graft and flow assessed before and after enhancement with papaverine. A resting flow below 100 ml, which does not double after papaverine, suggests that something is wrong. The best test is probably on-table angiography because it shows the anastomosis and also the run-off vessels. Any problem can then be seen and dealt with immediately. This technique is described in Chapter 3. If there is any doubt, the anastomosis should be opened. This is best done by unravelling the sutures down one side of the anastomosis back to the corners, this will give a good view of the interior and allow any remedial procedure to be performed. Once the graft has been re-sutured, a further arteriogram should be performed to ensure that the problem has been overcome.

DECISION POINTS OF THE OPERATION

1.   Should the long saphenous vein be used, or some other form of graft? In general, if the long saphenous vein is available it should be preserved for later use below the knee. Veins less than 4 mm in diameter should not be used.
2.   Should the operation be performed above or below the knee? If there is any doubt about the preoperative angiogram, then an on-table angiogram must be performed to assess the correct level of the distal anastomosis.
3.   Has the operation been successful? This can be answered as mentioned earlier by on-table angiography. Palpation of the pulses is also useful if they have been exposed sufficiently to allow access.

POSTOPERATIVE CARE

The patient will usually have lost only a little blood and a careful watch should be kept on the blood pressure and pulse. Hypotension during the postoperative period is one cause of early graft thrombosis. Because of the risk of associated myocardial ischaemia, the patient should be monitored for 24 hours. The pulses should be looked for and regularly felt and any bleeding noted. The drain should be removed within 24 hours and the patient encouraged to ambulate on the first postoperative day. Antibiotics should not be continued after 24 hours unless there is specific indication for doing so. If the patient has had an artificial graft inserted, there is some evidence that antiplatelet agents such as aspirin should be administered routinely.

INDICATIONS FOR RE-EXPLORATION

If the graft thromboses early, i.e. in the first 24–48 hours, and the indications at surgery were that a technically satisfactory procedure had been performed, the patient should be re-explored without delay. This requires proper general, or, if the patient's condition is poor, local anaesthesia, the provision of blood and the opening of both wounds. The distal anastomosis is opened along one side, a Fogarty catheter (no. 3) passed and the graft emptied of clot. Adequate flow will then occur down the graft. The distal anastomosis will have to be inspected carefully for any technical problem and, if none can be found, simply resutured. Further on-table arteriography should then be performed and the patient given heparin, which should be maintained postoperatively for 24 hours. If, at the time of the operation, the distal run-off was poorer than was thought to be the case, or if the risk was high, then it might be best not to re-explore as the chances of success would be poor. Alternatively, the graft may have to be inserted into a crural vessel.

RESULTS

The results of above-knee procedures are very good, the five-year patency rate being of the order of 70% for saphenous vein, diminishing to 30% with Dacron.[2] The results depend upon the run-off, patients with three vessel run-off doing better than those with two, who in turn do better than those with one. The operation provides very adequate limb salvage.

REFERENCES

1   Owen K, Rob C G 1956 Technique for bypass operations in femoral
      arterial disease. British Medical Journal 11: 273–275
2   Rutherford A B, Jones D N, Bergentz S E et al 1988 Factors affecting
      patency of infrainguinal bypass. Journal of Vascular Surgery 8:
      236–246
3   Garrett L, El-Dean S, Jordan C et al 1985 The pattern of arteriosclerotic
      changes in the peripheral arteries and the role of physical exercise.
      Alaska Medicine 55: 26–31
4   Quin R D, Evans D H, Bell P R F 1975 Haemodynamic assessment of
      the aortoiliac segment. Journal of Cardiovascular Surgery 16:
      586–589
5   Macpherson D S, Evans D H, Bell P R F 1984 Common femoral artery
      Doppler waveform: a comparison of three methods of objective
      analysis with direct pressure measurement. British Journal of Surgery
      71: 46–49
6   Quinones-Baldrick W J, Busuttil R W, Baker J D et al 1988 Is the
      preferential use of polytetrafluoroethylene grafts for femoropopliteal
      bypass justified? Journal of Vascular Surgery 8: 219–228
7   Harris P L, How T V, Jones D P 1987 Prospective randomised clinical
      trial to compare in situ and reversed saphenous vein grafts for
      femoropopliteal bypass. British Journal of Surgery 74: 252–254
8   Bagi P, Schroder T, Silleson H, Lorentzen J E 1989 Real time B mode
      mapping of the greater saphenous vein. European Journal of Vascular
      Surgery 3: 103–107
9   Moseley J G, Marston A 1986 A 5-year follow up of Dacron
      femoropopliteal bypass grafts. British Journal of Surgery 73: 24–28

Chapter 11

Femoropopliteal grafts below the knee

Introduction

This procedure is performed for obstruction to the femoral and popliteal artery where the occlusion extends beyond the knee joint, leaving a patent segment immediately above the trifurcation (Fig. 11.1). The results of surgery in this area are just as good, if not slightly better, than those of the above knee procedure.[1] The patient's own long saphenous vein provides the best results, but if this is not available and the procedure is being done for limb salvage, then other forms of grafts such as PTFE, Dacron or human umbilical vein can be used. The only controlled trial so far done suggests that human umbilical vein gives the best results.[2] However, it is prone to aneurysm formation with the passage of time. At this level the long saphenous vein is often narrow and controversy exists as to whether the vein used in situ is preferable to its removal and reversal. Recent published results would suggest that there is no difference between these two procedures.[3] In general, however, the in situ procedure is preferable because it allows the smaller distal end of the vein to be stitched to the smaller distal vessels, especially if the crural arteries are being revascularised. Haemodynamically the results are probably the same.[4]

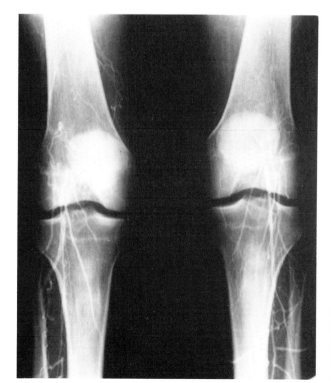

Fig. 11.1
Femoropopliteal obstruction with a patent below-knee popliteal artery suitable for a below-knee femoropopliteal graft on either side.

EXPOSURE OF THE FEMORAL ARTERY IN THE GROIN

This should be undertaken in exactly the same way as already described for a femoropopliteal graft placed above the knee. The incision can be either vertical or oblique (Fig. 11.2) and the femoral artery with the profunda femoris and its first two branches should be exposed. Silastic slings should then be placed around these vessels (Fig. 11.3). The upper branches of the long saphenous vein should be exposed, along with the saphenofemoral junction (Fig. 11.4).

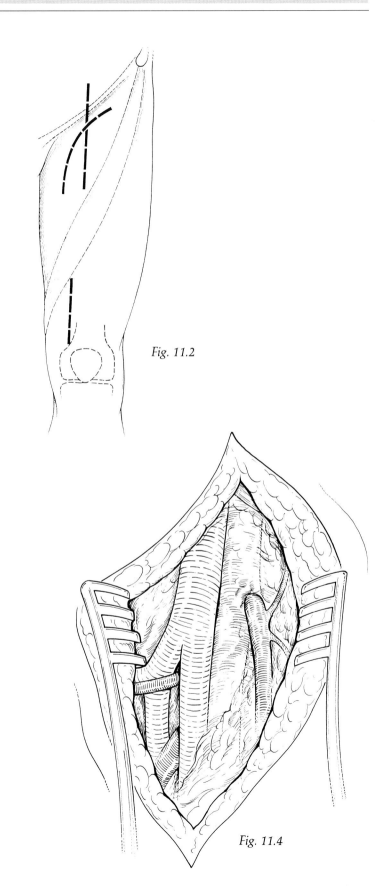

Fig. 11.2

Fig. 11.3

Fig. 11.4

EXPOSURE OF THE POPLITEAL TRIFURCATION

The limb is bent at an angle of about 40° and an incision made along the medial border of the leg behind the tibia, the upper end curving backwards along the gastrocnemius muscle (Fig. 11.5). Care should be taken when making this incision not to damage the long saphenous vein, which will usually be seen at the anterior edge of the wound. If a Duplex machine is available, preoperative mapping and marking of the vein will be a great help.[5] Having cut through the superficial fascia and fat, the deep fascia will next be encountered and the gastrocnemius muscle seen immediately behind it. A longitudinal incision is now made in the deep fascia immediately behind the tibia (Fig. 11.6). Once this fascia is divided, the gastrocnemius muscle tends to fall back revealing the soleus and its attachment to the tibia. By retracting the upper edge of the wound, the femoral artery and vein can usually be seen and certainly felt just before they pass underneath the soleus and gastrocnemius muscles. Using a pair of artery forceps and curved scissors, the fascia overlying the vessels is now divided and right-angled forceps introduced under the soleus muscle immediately in front of the vessels and nerves. The muscle is now divided as shown in Figure 11.7, close to its attachment to the tibia.

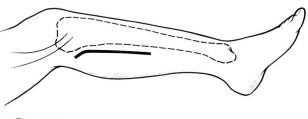

Fig. 11.5

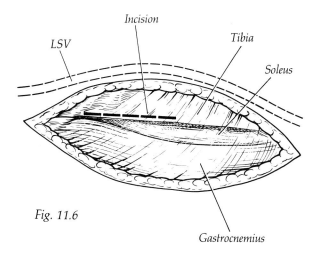

Fig. 11.6

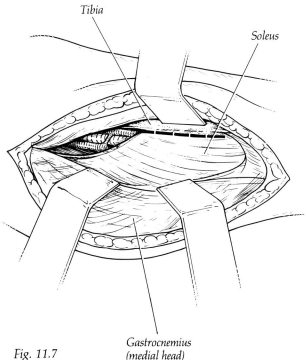

Fig. 11.7

Division of this muscle continues downwards until the popliteal artery is exposed with its various branches. This usually means separating about 5 cm of the muscle from the tibia. Some bleeding occurs from small vessels which can be dealt with by diathermy or ligature (Fig. 11.8). The neurovascular bundle will now be seen in the depths of the wound and the artery is difficult to separate from the veins, which are very closely applied to it. The popliteal vein usually covers the artery and there are numerous intercommunicating veins criss-crossing the popliteal artery and its branches. These vessels bleed a great deal and have to be ligated. The first step is to incise the fascia overlying the main popliteal artery, which can usually by now be seen, and divide it carefully isolating a small segment of the vessel. If the vein is in the way, this should first of all be encircled and controlled with a silastic sling. Be careful not to damage the vein which is very closely applied to the artery. Patience will be rewarded with success. Once the artery has been isolated, a right-angled clamp is placed around it and a silastic sling placed as in Figure 11.9. Once this sling has been placed, by exerting gentle traction on it in a direction away from the tibia, the anterior tibial artery will be seen—at least its origin—as it passes towards the interosseous membrane. This vessel can now be encircled in a similar way using a right-angled clamp if it appears to be easy—if not, leave it alone (Fig. 11.10).

The main tibioperoneal trunk can now be followed downwards keeping close to the arterial wall with scissors. As each communicating vein is encountered, it should be carefully divided between ligatures as in Figures 11.11 and 11.12. These veins cannot be diathermised satisfactorily and once they slip out of sight can be difficult to find again.

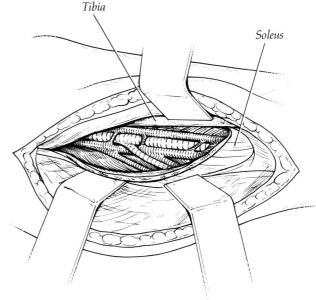

Fig. 11.8

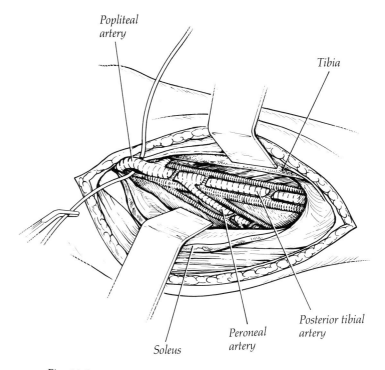

Fig. 11.9

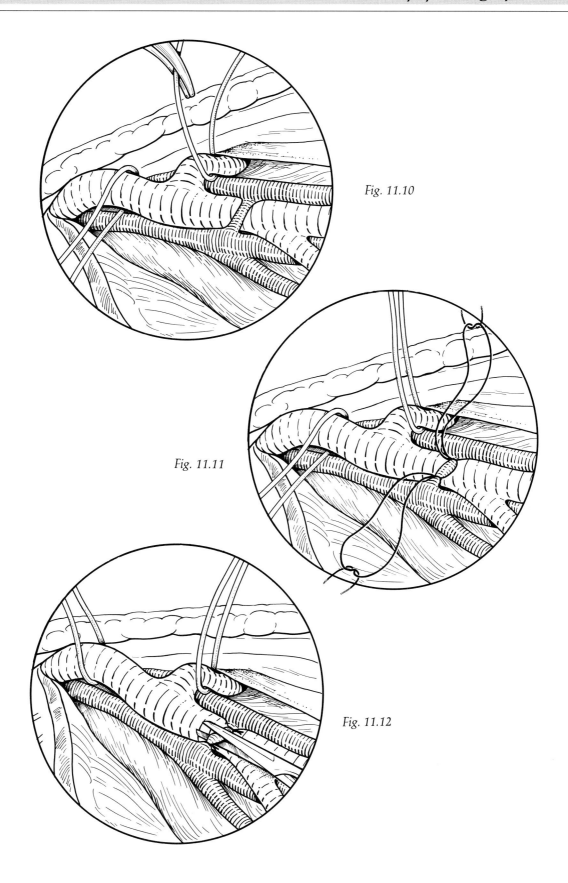

Fig. 11.10

Fig. 11.11

Fig. 11.12

Divide as many veins as are necessary to see the arteries properly. After dividing two or three such veins, the tibioperoneal trunk will be seen, as in Figure 11.13, which then divides into the posterior tibial artery and the peroneal artery. Again, any veins in front of these vessels are carefully ligated and divided. Sometimes it is difficult to decide which is the posterior tibial artery and which is the peroneal artery. The latter usually passes more posteriorly, but on-table arteriography may be necessary to make the final decision about this point. Now that the vessels are exposed, slings should be placed around the posterior tibial and peroneal arteries as in Figure 11.13. A decision needs to be made about where the graft is to be placed. If arteriography indicates that the main popliteal artery is patent, then it may be sufficient to simply place the graft as high as possible proximal to the anterior tibial artery, although this is sometimes difficult. If access is difficult, or the graft

appears to be compressed by them, the tendons of Gracilis and semitendinosus can be cut. The incision into the artery can be made either above the anterior tibial artery or below it in the tibio-peroneal trunk, as shown in Figure 11.14. Whichever site is chosen will depend on examination of the pre-operative angiogram, or an on-table arteriogram done immediately before progressing any further. Before the arteriotomy is made, a soft vascular clamp should be placed proximally. The branches of the artery can usually be controlled by gentle traction on the slings around them—this avoids damage to calcified or small vessels. If this is not possible, or it does not result in reasonable control, vascular clamps can be placed across the soft non-calcified parts of the artery or a Fogarty catheter inflated inside the vessel and kept inflated by attachment to a three-way tap. If an in situ vein graft is to be used, then the operation will proceed as described for that technique later in this

book. If, however, a reversed vein graft is to be used, then the vein must be removed through either a continuous incision or multiple incisions, as described for the femoropopliteal operation above the knee. If that method is chosen, the incision must be made carefully so as to avoid damage to the vein, making sure that an adequate length is removed. If an artificial graft or reversed saphenous vein is being used, a tunnel must next be made between the lower and upper incisions. This is done by passing a tunnelling instrument from below upwards: the tunneller is placed immediately superficial to the popliteal artery and then passed along it gently. As the instrument passes above the knee joint it has to be angled in a super-ficial direction to pass towards the anterior compartment of the thigh, emerging at the groin. If this proves difficult, the instrument should be passed from above downwards, again starting close to the femoral artery and emerging at the lower wound close to

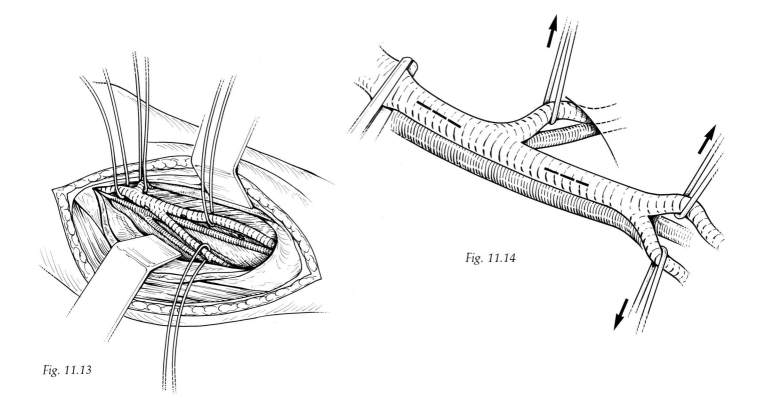

Fig. 11.13

Fig. 11.14

the popliteal. This is best done with the leg straight (Fig. 11.15). Once the tunneller has been passed, the obturator is removed and a long pair of forceps passed along the tunneller to grasp the graft as described in the previous section. Once the graft has passed through the tunneller, its proximal end is held and the tunnelling tool removed. The upper or lower anastomosis is next constructed in an end-to-side fashion in exactly the same way as described for femoral popliteal grafts above the knee. The lower end of an externally supported PTFE graft is shown being sutured to the popliteal artery in Figure 11.16. In general, as the patient is heparinised, it is better to construct the lower anastomosis first with the knee bent. Once this has been done, and ensuring that the graft is not twisted by allowing free back-bleeding to occur, the leg is straightened. This allows the correct length of graft to be estimated and excess removed. The upper

anastomosis can then be completed. If the upper anastomosis is constructed first it has the advantage that forward flow can be tested on its completion. The exact amount of graft necessary, with the leg straightened, has to be cut and the leg then bent to complete the anastomosis. The anastomoses are constructed in the same manner as described for an above-knee femoropopliteal graft. Once again, before final sutures are inserted back and forward bleeding are assessed. Completion angiography is important after the graft has been inserted to ensure that the procedure is satisfactory.

PROBLEMS DURING THE OPERATION

These should be few in number. It is important to get the length of the graft correct and avoid too little or too much tension. In the former case, unsupported

graft will kink easily and in the latter the anastomosis can be adversely affected. Be careful not to construct the lower anastomosis with the leg bent unless you have first of all ensured that the length of the graft required is sufficient for it to be easily straightened later.

RESULTS

The results of this procedure are very good and, provided long saphenous vein is used, are similar to those that can be expected for above-knee procedures, with a five-year patency of 65%.[1] The eventual result will, of course, depend upon run-off: with a three-vessel run-off the results are best, but with a single vessel run-off they are proportionally worse. If there is a single vessel run-off into the calf in direct continuation with the popliteal artery, it is usually best to insert a graft into the popliteal artery rather than into the crural artery lower down the leg.

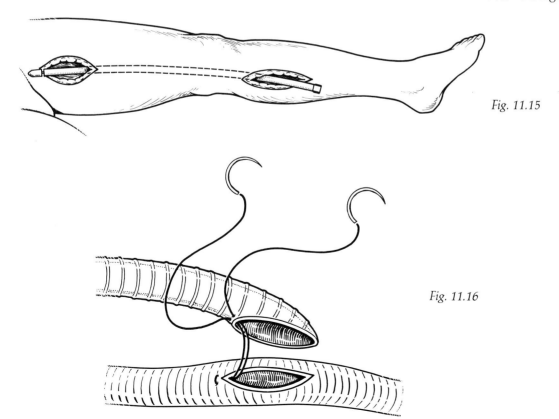

Fig. 11.15

Fig. 11.16

REFERENCES

1   Rutherford R B, Jones D N, Bergentz S E et al 1988 Factors affecting the
      patency of infrainguinal bypass. Journal of Vascular Surgery 8:
      236–246
2   Aicknoff J H, Buchardt Hansen H J, Bromme A et al 1983 A randomised
      clinical trial of PTFE versus human umbilical vein for femoropopliteal
      bypass surgery. Preliminary results. British Journal of Surgery 70:
      85–89
3   Watelet J, Chacysson E, Poels D, Menhard J F, Papion H, Testart S N
      1986 In situ versus reversed saphenous vein for femoropopliteal
      bypass. A prospective randomised study of 100 cases. Annals of
      Vascular Surgery 1: 441–452
4   Beard J D, Lee R E, Aldoori M I, Baird R N, Horrocks M 1986 Does the
      in situ technique for autologous vein femoropopliteal bypass offer
      any haemodynamic advantage? Journal of Vascular Surgery 4:
      564–588
5   Bagi P, Schroder T, Silleson H, Lorentzen J E 1989 Real time B mode
      mapping of the greater saphenous vein. European Journal of Vascular
      Surgery 3: 103–107

Chapter 12

In situ saphenous vein bypass grafting

Introduction

This technique was described some years ago, but only recently has its popularity become firmly established. Although first described by Rob[1] as a potentially quicker way of doing a bypass procedure, it was popularised by Hall[2] who first described a successful method of rendering the venous valves incompetent. The procedure was thought to have a number of potential advantages over and above the reversed saphenous vein graft. These included better viability of the vein as its blood supply was relatively undisturbed, better haemodynamics (the wide end to the vein being at the top, and the narrow end distally) and also that smaller veins could be used. With the exception of the last statement, there is no evidence that in situ vein grafting holds any advantages over the reversed operation except distally in the lower leg. Recent publications have in fact suggested that the reversed procedure produces equally good results to in situ grafting when used to the popliteal artery either above or below the knee.[3] With this in mind and remembering that this operation often takes longer, it should probably not be used above the knee. Its main place is for grafting to the distal popliteal artery below the knee or to one of the tibial or peroneal vessels in the calf or at the ankle. Saphenous vein used in the in situ fashion produces the best results for distal surgery and should be used as a first choice in this position.[4] Apart from tapering in the right direction, it offers no haemodynamic advantage.[5] The operation is quite difficult and technically demanding, requires time and, without proper care, can produce poor results.

INDICATIONS

Below-knee femoropopliteal or femorocrural grafting for severe < 50-yard claudication or critical ischaemia.

OPERATION

The patient usually requires general or spinal anaesthesia and an operative time of approximately three hours should be allowed. Various incisions are acceptable. The vein can be mobilised through a series of vertical incisions, maintaining bridges of skin in between, or alternatively a continuous incision from groin to the distal vessel can be used (Fig. 12.1). My personal preference is for the latter because it allows the vein to be properly exposed, all branches to be ligated and, most importantly, allows the operator to see the valve stripper and feel it as it passes down the vein, thereby avoiding undue damage. Starting above, the incision is deepened as already described for femoropopliteal grafting, to expose the femoral artery, its two main branches and the long saphenous vein (Fig. 12.2). Dissection should be carried down to the first two branches of the profunda femoris and slings passed as shown to control this vessel along with the common and superficial femoral arteries, as described for femoropopliteal bypass (Fig. 12.3). The long saphenous vein, which has already been exposed at its upper end, can be followed down for a few centimetres and preserved. The below-knee part of the incision should now be deepened and the popliteal artery and its trifurcation exposed, as previously described for below-knee femoropopliteal grafts. The reason for doing

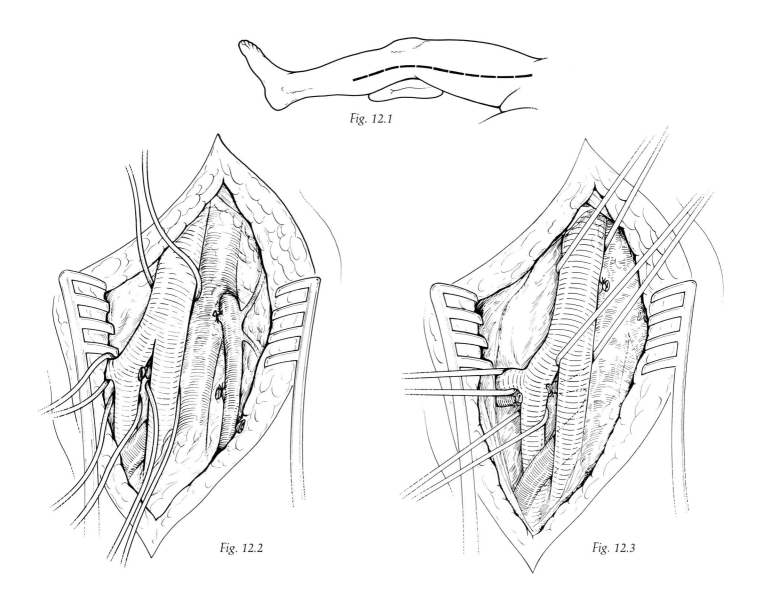

Fig. 12.1

Fig. 12.2

Fig. 12.3

this is to ensure that the operation is feasible and that the exact location for distal insertion of the vein is known prior to exposing it. Once the trifurcation has been exposed (Fig. 12.4 and see p. 132), unless preoperative arteriography is of a quality which allows distal definition, then an on-table arteriogram should be performed by inserting a needle into the popliteal artery and injecting contrast medium to obtain a good picture of the available vessels (see p. 28). This will allow the operator to plan exactly where the distal anastomosis should be. If the arteriogram confirms that the popliteal artery is the vessel of choice, then no more needs to be done at this stage. If, however, the anterior tibial, peroneal or posterior tibial is chosen, further dissection of these vessels as described on pages 164, 166, 170, will be necessary.

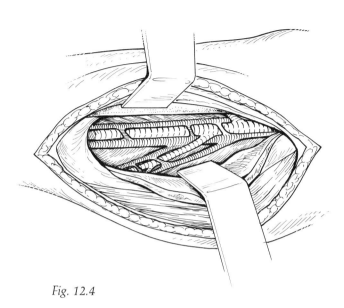

Fig. 12.4

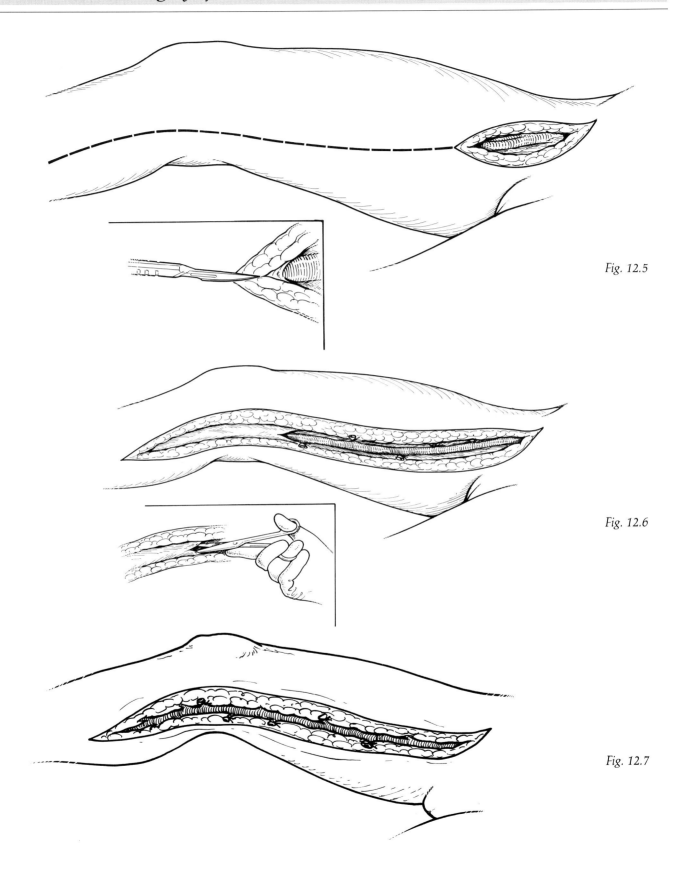

Fig. 12.5

Fig. 12.6

Fig. 12.7

Having established the distal limits of the procedure, the long saphenous vein is now exposed in its entirety. Starting in the groin, the vessel is followed downwards, dividing the skin little by little and the fascia around the vein with scissors as shown in Figures 12.5 and 12.6. In this way the vein will be completely displayed from the groin to the lower incision (Fig. 12.7). Great care should be taken distally as the vein is usually very close to the skin. Once the vein has been exposed, all the branches should be ligated in continuity using a non-absorbable ligature such as Neurolon or silk. A large branch of the vein is often seen in the upper third of the thigh—this should not be ligated until the vein is seen in its entirety as it

may peter out near the knee. In this event, the large branch will need to be followed to see if this is usable as an alternative. At this stage the patient is usually heparinised and the saphenous vein can be detached from its femoral insertion after deciding exactly where on the artery it will be sutured. It is often difficult to stretch the vein to reach the artery and it is important that tension should be avoided at the upper anastomosis. Usually, by dividing the upper two or three branches, it is

possible to swing the vein across without too much difficulty. As far as the lower end of the vein is concerned, its size is relatively unimportant as almost any size down to 2 mm is usable.

Options for upper anastomosis
A vascular clamp should be placed on the femoral vein (Fig. 12.8) to allow the saphenous vein, along with a small piece of femoral vein, to be removed. This gives extra length, but care must be taken not to narrow the femoral vein,

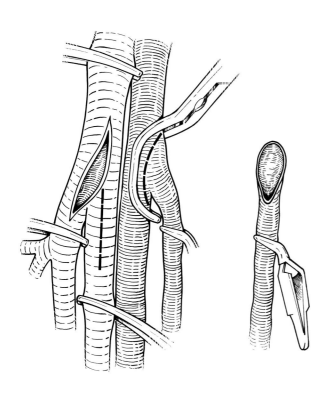

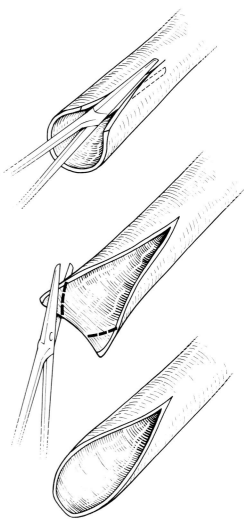

Fig. 12.8

Fig. 12.9

which must then be carefully oversewn with continuous 5/0 Prolene. An arteriotomy should then be made, preferably to incorporate the mouth of the profunda femoris artery, or alternatively extended across the origin of the superficial femoral artery. The vein is next prepared for anastomosis by cutting along one side (Fig. 12.9). The incision should match the arteriotomy and should usually be about 1 cm in length.

At this point, using a pair of fine atraumatic forceps, the superior saphenous valve should be grasped and excised as this is often difficult to destroy with the stripper later (Fig. 12.10). The vein should now be anastomosed to the femoral artery using 5/0 Prolene, two double-ended sutures being used at the heel and the toe, as shown in Figure 12.11. Once these are tied, one side of the anastomosis should be completed (Fig. 12.12) and the other

side stitched in such a way that the final knot is tied at the midpoint of the anastomosis (Fig. 12.13). As usual before completion, back bleeding from all branches and forward bleeding should be tested and any debris and clot removed. Another method of constructing the anastomosis is to use a single stitch inserted at the heel of the anastomosis and taken along each side, as described on page 122.

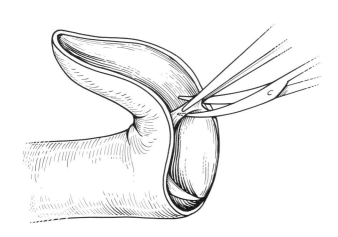

Fig. 12.10

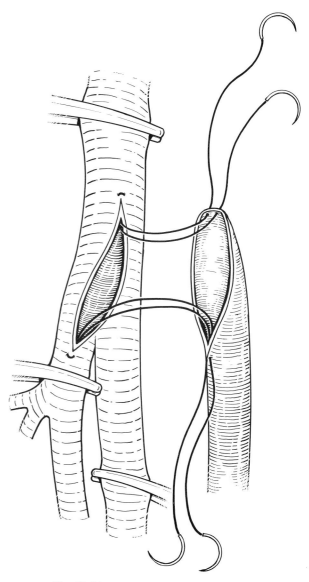

Fig. 12.11

Difficulties with the length of saphenous vein

Sometimes the saphenous vein is not long enough to reach the artery without using undue tension. Under these circumstances one of the following can be considered.

1. *Using a piece of the superficial femoral artery*. This will often be blocked, but an appropriate length can be chosen to allow no tension on the vein and the vessel divided as in Figure 12.14. It will then be necessary to remove the atheroma from inside the vessel by inserting an appropriate instrument, such as a Watson Cheyne dissector, passing it between the atheroma and the vessel wall in an appropriate plane.

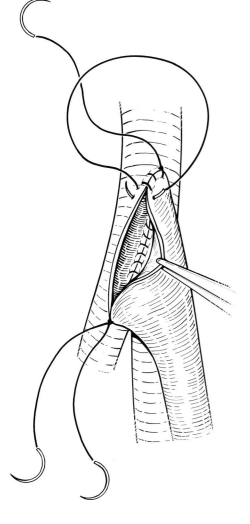

Fig. 12.12

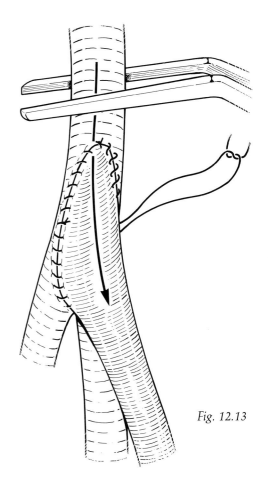

Fig. 12.13

Once the atheromatous material has been freed, it can be pulled out with a pair of artery forceps until good forward bleeding occurs. The atheroma generally splits across at the bifurcation and allows a good flow of blood distally. Once this has been done, the vein can then be sutured end-to-end with the endarterectomised artery as described on page 28; again 5/0 Prolene should be used (Fig. 12.15). This option is probably the least attractive of those available as the superficial femoral artery is prone to further development of atheroma.

2.   *Using a branch of the long saphenous vein.* Occasionally, a suitable branch is present passing superiorly from the long saphenous vein medial to its insertion. This can be of sufficient calibre to allow the anastomosis to be made to the femoral artery without tension. Generally, however, this branch is quite small and this alternative is not a satisfactory one (Fig. 12.16).

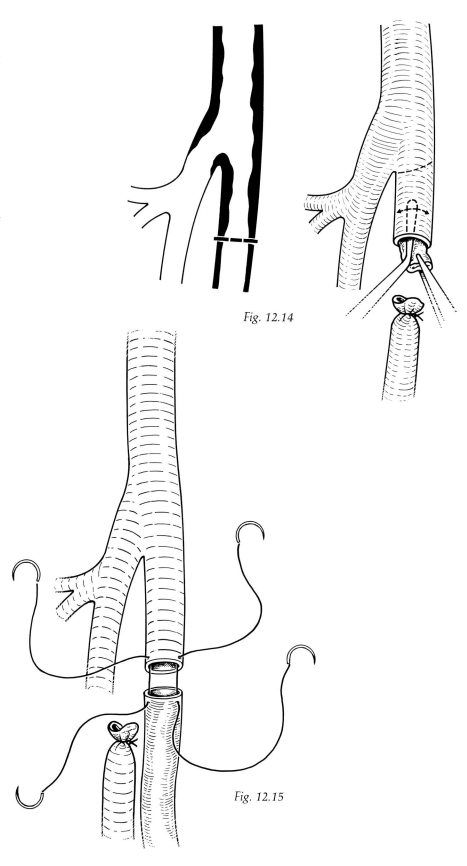

Fig. 12.14

Fig. 12.15

3.   *Use of an additional segment of vein.* Sometimes a large branch of the long saphenous vein appears in the thigh as previously mentioned and, if this is not for use in the operation, a piece of it can be excised, reversed and stitched on to the end of the long saphenous vein to allow it to reach the femoral vein with ease. If this is not possible, however, then a piece of cephalic vein from either arm should be removed and provides an excellent substitute (Fig. 12.17). In this event, the segment of vein should be stitched end-to-end with the existing saphenous vein, using interrupted 6/0 Prolene (see p. 28) and then anastomosed, as already described on page 120, to the femoral artery at the chosen site. The alternative, using a piece of Goretex to form a composite graft at the upper end, is not to be recommended.

4.   *Non-reversed in situ bypass.* Another way of getting the vein to reach the artery is to use it as an in situ graft, thereby taking advantage of the taper, but to mobilise it completely by dividing all branches so that it can slide up and down the leg. By taking more of the distal vein, it can be slid proximally and easily reach the artery. Used in this way good results can be obtained.[8]

Using one of these methods, it is usually possible to attach the long saphenous vein to the femoral artery at its upper end as already described for femoro-popliteal bypass grafting. Whichever technique is used, the superior valve must first be excised as already described. The distal limit of the vein is now decided upon, having straightened the leg first to get the length right. When this has been done, the vein is divided and the distal end tied. The clamps are now released and arterial blood will be seen to pass down the vein and stop at the first valve beyond the one already excised. The distal part of the vein is now gently grasped and the smallest valvulotome (2 mm) selected, inserted carefully and pushed proximally (Fig. 12.18).

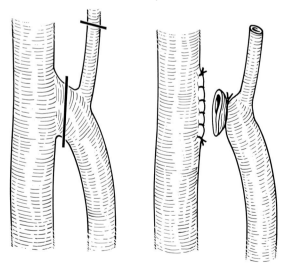

Fig. 12.16

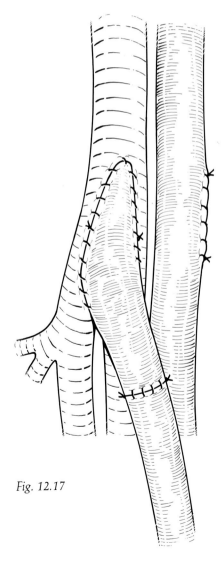

Fig. 12.17

It is important to watch the progress of the stripper and to palpate it throughout the length of the vein (Fig. 12.19). When the stripper reaches the upper end, it is then gently withdrawn using a circular movement to do so and in no circumstances using undue traction. As each valve is encountered the finger of the opposite hand is placed on the vein while the stripper is gently removed with a twisting movement. As each valve is passed, blood passes down to the next one. Eventually the stripper is withdrawn and pulsatile arterial bleeding should occur (Fig. 12.20). The stripper should be passed at least once more to ensure that adequate bleeding occurs, as once the lower anastomosis is completed it is difficult to pass the stripper. The vein is now clamped close to the proximal anastomosis using a soft vascular clamp.

An alternative method of destroying the valves is to leave the vein attached at the saphenofemoral junction and divide it distally. The chosen valvulotome can then be passed from below upwards and gently withdrawn until venous blood refluxes freely down the vein. The upper and lower anastomosis can then be completed in whichever order is the preference of the surgeon.[6]

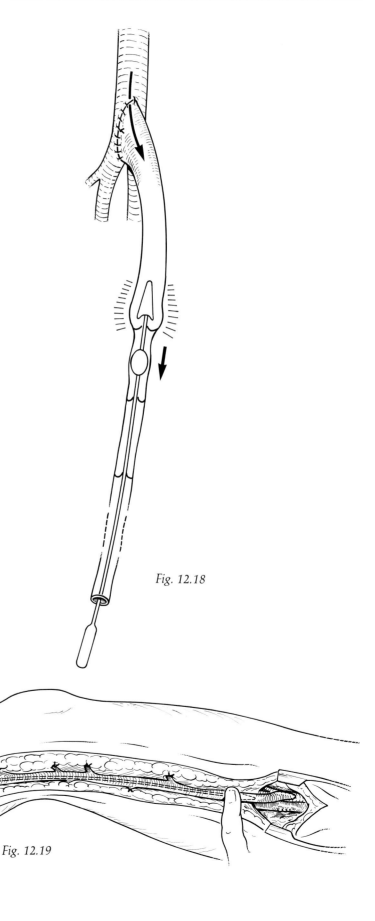

Fig. 12.18

Fig. 12.19

An arteriotomy is then made at the chosen site in the lower vessel (Fig. 12.21), the leg straightened and the vein adjusted to its final length, bearing in mind it has to pass from a superficial position into the depths of the wound. Make sure it is not twisted. The vein is divided and cut along one side as previously described on page 142. The knee can now be bent again to facilitate access to the popliteal artery. The anastomosis is now completed using two 6/0 Prolene sutures or a single one at the heel as described on page 120 (Fig. 12.22).

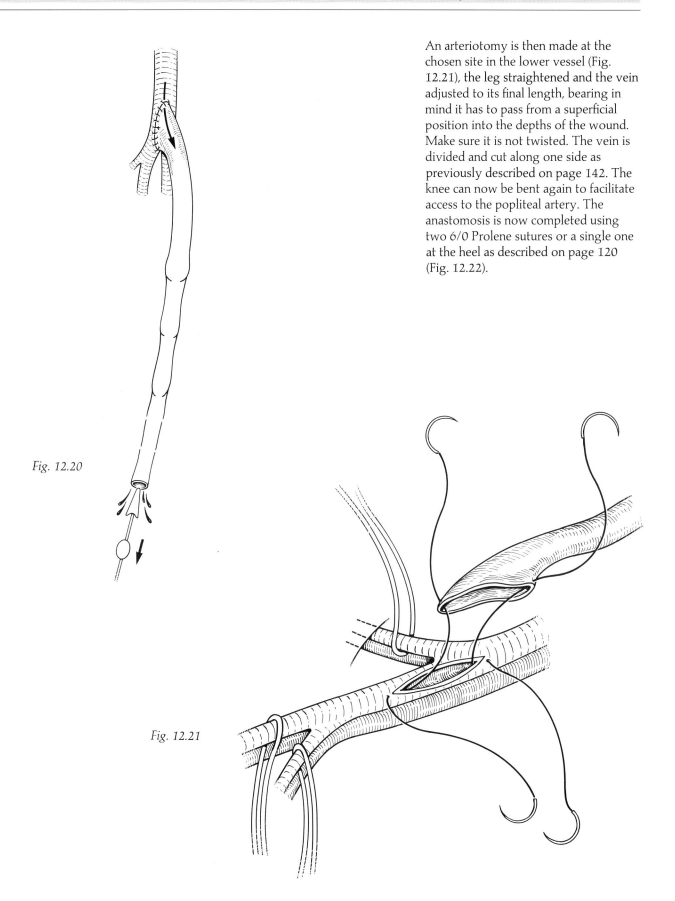

Fig. 12.20

Fig. 12.21

For more distal anastomoses it is important to use interrupted sutures at the toe of the anastomosis, depending upon its size (Figs 12.23 and 12.24). A magnifying loupe is important if technical errors are to be avoided. The clamps are now finally released, the leg straightened and a careful examination made to ensure that the vein is not kinked as it passes to the depths of the wound.

The valvulotome described here is the original one described by Hall. Several other types (Fig. 12.25) have been used, including the cutting valvulotome and scissors popularised by Karmody and Leather[7] and, more recently, a disposable type with a following balloon. In my experience, the Hall's stripper used carefully at its smallest diameter is satisfactory, but the new disposable ones will probably be better.

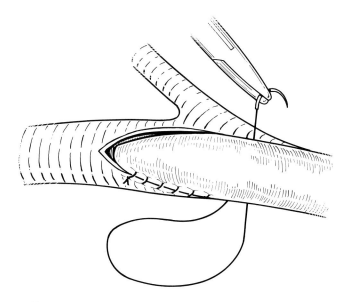

Fig. 12.22

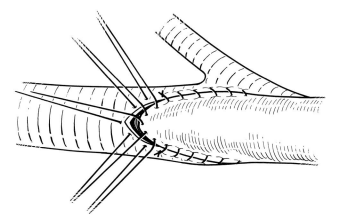

Fig. 12.23

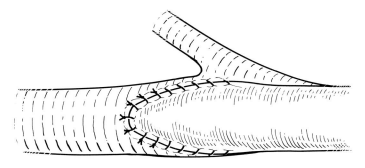

Fig. 12.24

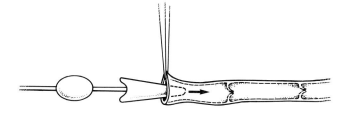

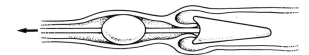

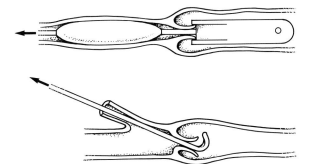

Ensuring all branches are tied
There are several ways of doing this. The best one is probably arteriography. By using two films and two injections it is also possible to see the distal anastomosis, which is essential in any case after completing surgery. Artery forceps or clips are used to mark the levels (Fig. 12.26) and contrast injected into the graft after clamping it proximally with a vascular clamp. Any branches are easily seen and can then be tied. Moving the plate lower down the leg, a second film will demonstrate the distal anastomosis (Fig. 12.27). If there are any doubts about the anastomosis it should be reopened and refashioned as described on page 123. Patent branches can also be located by placing a flow meter around the vein graft and clamping it at intervals from above downwards. If there is no flow all branches have been tied, if flow occurs there is a branch between the clamp and the proximal anastomosis. Another technique is to look for branches prior to completing the lower anastomosis.

Fig. 12.25

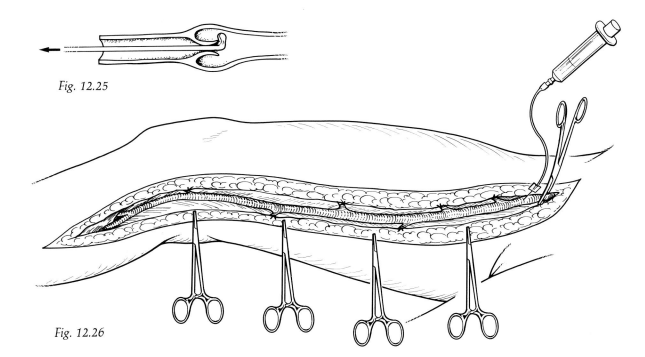

Fig. 12.26

After completing the upper anastomosis a clamp is placed across the vein near to its lower end and heparinised saline injected gently from below. If the saline can be injected then a branch must be present and is looked for, if not the clamp is moved successively upwards until it reaches the top. Any of these techniques are acceptable but an arteriogram, as mentioned earlier, probably provides the best and most direct method of seeing what is happening. If all is well, the wound is closed in layers, using catgut to the fat to ensure appropriate apposition of the edges and continuous or interrupted fine sutures to the skin—nylon or metal skin clips are best. A drain should be inserted at both ends, passing along the vein upwards and downwards to allow adequate drainage for 24 hours.

DECISION POINTS OF THE OPERATION

The most obvious problems relate to the vein and to the site of the distal anastomosis. The vein should not be divided until the operator is certain where the distal anastomosis is going to be. If the vein is inadequate, i.e. below 2 mm, then another branch should be looked for or an alternative sought. At the upper end one of the alternatives suggested should be used and there should be no difficulty in getting adequate length. On no account should the vein be stretched or the graft will not work. When the valves are being destroyed or rendered incompetent it is vital that excessive force is not used when each valve cusp is encountered. Do not use the largest stripper possible, the smallest one that will enter the vein comfortably should be used and used with care otherwise intimal stripping and destruction of the vein will be the result (Fig. 12.28).

RESULTS

As mentioned previously, there is probably no difference between an in situ procedure and the reversed operation above or immediately below the knee.[3] However, for distal procedures to the peroneal artery or the tibials an in situ vein graft provides better results than the alternatives available, such as human umbilical vein or PTFE, and should not be used in this location. Because vein provides the best results at this site it should probably not be used higher up, being reserved for later distal bypass if required.

An advantage of the in situ operation is that, because of the subcutaneous location of the vessel, it is usually possible to follow its progress by repeated Duplex scanning. If surveillance suggests a problem is occurring then arteriography and corrective action can be taken easily and before the graft thromboses.

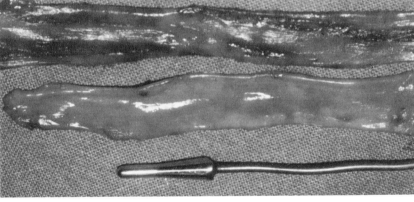

Fig. 12.28
Careless use of the valvulotome can cause irreversible damage to the vein.

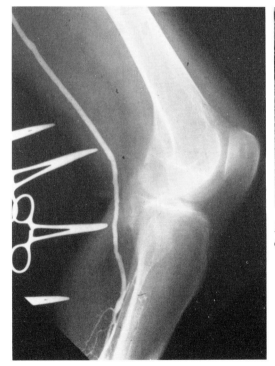

Fig. 12.27
On-table completion arteriogram after in situ vein grafting. The artery forceps act as markers for branches. In this case there are no branches untied and the distal anastomosis looks satisfactory.

REFERENCES

1　Rob C G, Eastcott H H G, Owen K 1956 The reconstruction of the arteries. British Journal of Surgery 43: 449–453
2　Hall K V 1962 The great saphenous vein used in situ as an arterial shunt after exterpation of vein valves. Surgery 51: 49–95
3　Harris P L, How T V, Jones D P 1987 Prospective randomised clinical trial to compare in situ and reversed saphenous vein grafts for femoropopliteal bypass. British Journal of Surgery 74: 252
4　Rutherford R B, Jones D N, Bergentz S E et al 1988 Factors affecting the patency of infrainguinal bypass. Journal of Vascular Surgery 8: 236–246
5　Beard J D, Lee R E, Aldori M I, Baird R N, Horrocks M 1986 Does the in situ technique for autologous vein femoropopliteal bypass offer any haemodynamic advantage? Journal of Vascular Surgery 4: 588–594
6　Gruss J D 1983 Technische aspektes des femoro-poplitealen und femoro-cruralen in situ bypass. Angiology 5: 49–53
7　Leather R P, Corson J D, Karmody A M 1984 Instrumental evolution of the valve incision method of in situ vein bypass. Journal of Vascular Surgery 1: 113–116
8　Beard J D, Wyatt M, Scott D J A, Baird R N, Horrocks M 1989 The non-reversed vein femorodistal bypass graft: a modification of the standard in situ technique. European Journal of Vascular Surgery 3(1): 55–61

Chapter 13

Femoral distal (crural) grafts

Introduction

Grafts to the lower limb vessels, namely the tibial or peroneal arteries, are usually done in order to save the leg from amputation. This procedure should not usually be performed on patients with claudication as the results in the long term can be poor.[1]

However, in the group of patients normally seen with this problem, namely elderly people who have a short life expectancy, this procedure is useful in order to try and avoid an amputation.

INDICATIONS

The patient, as already mentioned, will usually be relatively elderly and will present with rest pain and early gangrene of one or more toes. Examination of the limb will reveal that there are no pulses beyond the femoral and severe clinical ischaemia will be obvious. Investigations will usually reveal a normal inflow, no obvious profunda stenosis and an arteriogram which shows either an absence of distal vessels or, at best, a single vessel in the calf or lower regions of the leg. The X-ray findings can be confirmed by measuring the ankle pressure, which should be below 50 mmHg in order to comply with the currently accepted criteria for critical ischaemia.[2] The Doppler can be used to identify forward flow in any of the three ankle arteries, with the leg dependent, to see whether this agrees with the arteriographic findings. If the arteriogram shows no vessels at all (Fig. 13.1), this does not mean there are none present and a prelude to any procedure of this type is an angiogram performed at the time of surgery.

In such patients the important points are first of all to assess inflow and, if in doubt, to do a papaverine test to make certain that it is acceptable (see p. 5). If there is an inflow problem, deal with it by angioplasty or by surgery first as this will often solve the problem. If there is no inflow deficit then the next question will be, is there a reasonable distal vessel to which the graft can be attached? As already mentioned, a pre-operative angiogram is often of little value for this purpose. The vessels below the knee can be examined with a simple Doppler probe after hanging the legs over the bed and listening for a signal. Alternatively, pressure generated run-off (PGR) (Fig. 13.2) can be employed (see p. 7). This entails putting a cuff around the upper calf and rapidly inflating and deflating it to produce a signal which can be heard at the ankle by Doppler and given a score.[3] With this information available, the appropriate vessel can be explored either in the calf or near the ankle and an on-table angiogram with resistance measurements made as described later in this chapter and also in Chapter 2. If the saphenous vein is not available, or if the resistance is above 1400 mPRU, the chances of success are poor and a primary amputation should be considered.[4]

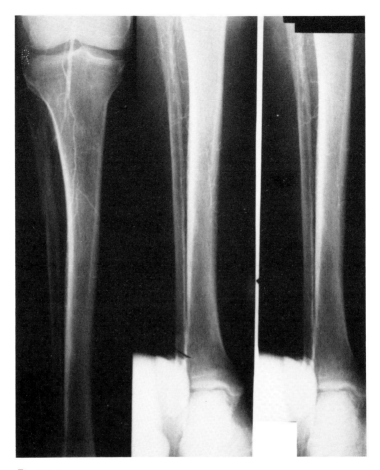

Fig. 13.1

Preoperative angiogram of a patient with critical ischaemia. No distal vessels are shown—although this does not mean that there are none.

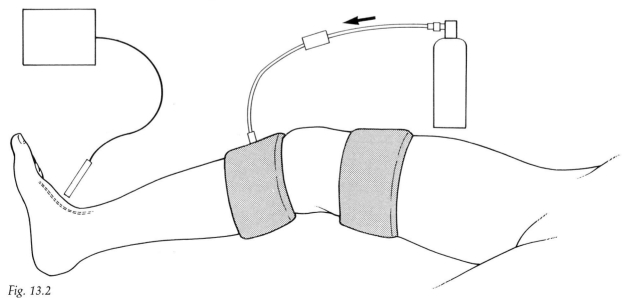

Fig. 13.2

Measuring pressure generated run-off (PGR). A cuff is placed as shown and intermittently inflated and deflated, producing a signal at the ankle which can be heard by Doppler at the ankle indicating that the vessel is patent.

USE OF AUTOLOGOUS VEIN

Although the long saphenous vein is usually the vessel of choice, this may not always be available and, as veins give the best results particularly for distal vessels, efforts should be made to try and assess its adequacy prior to surgical intervention. If facilities are available, Duplex mapping,[5] or the use of non-ionic contrast for saphenous venography, will show the vein and allow its quality to be assessed. If the vein is judged to be deficient, before considering artificial grafts it is important to remember that other veins can be used, such as the short saphenous vein which passes down the middle of the lower leg and is often available. The cephalic vein or basilic vein in the arm can also be used without difficulty (Fig. 13.3). The latter is particularly useful if it can be removed with the cephalic vein, as the two are often joined at the elbow. The basilic element can be used as an in situ graft with destruction of the valves, and its continuation, the cephalic vein, can be used without interference to the valves. In this way, a long secondary vein useful for below the knee obstructions can be obtained.[6] The veins are removed through multiple or continuous incisions in exactly the same way as described earlier (Ch. 10) for the long saphenous vein. Arm veins, however, are usually thinner and great care must be taken in handling them. The wounds in the arm usually heal without any problems.

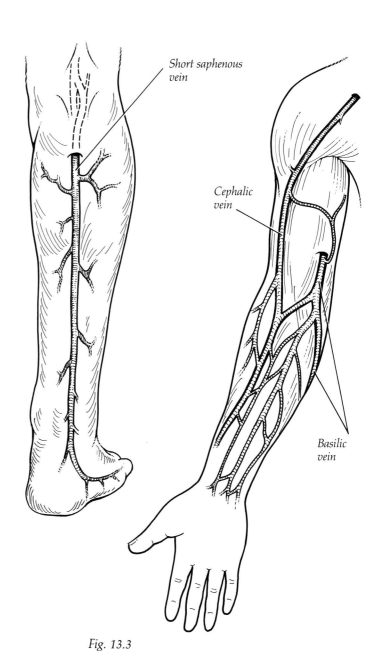

Short saphenous vein

Cephalic vein

Basilic vein

Fig. 13.3

PREOPERATIVE PREPARATION

Apart from the usual preparations for any vascular procedure, already described in Chapter 1, in these patients there are other problems. Often they are in poor cardiac and respiratory condition and the help of an experienced physician is important to give the best chances of success. Similarly, an experienced anaesthetist will be able to take the patient safely through the procedure. An additional problem in these patients is the presence of severe infection, which will increase the chances of wound and graft infection. For this reason, a wide spectrum of antibiotics should be given and continued for a full postoperative course of treatment. Good cover is obtained with cloxacillin, gentamicin and metronidazole, but care must be taken to ensure that renal toxicity does not occur and levels of gentamicin must be measured regularly. Diabetics need to have their disease controlled and insulin is usually required for this purpose.

INTRAOPERATIVE INVESTIGATIONS PRIOR TO FEMORODISTAL GRAFTING

There is no quantitative method of accurately deciding which patients will do well after this type of operation. Some patients experience useful limb salvage, which has to be aimed for in this high-risk group, but on the other hand there is little point in performing an expensive, time-consuming operation which is doomed to fail and expose the patient to a later amputation which might be at a higher level.[7] In view of this, a number of centres have been measuring the peripheral resistance of the outflow tract before deciding about the advisability of surgery. If the resistance is high, then this is generally speaking a bad sign. Ascer et al[8] have measured resistance using saline following completion of the anastomosis and suggest that the outcome can be related to this measurement. We have measured the resistance before doing the operation in order to decide if reconstruction is worthwhile.[4] Resistance is not the only important factor, but the existence of too many risk factors should suggest that the patient would be better served by primary amputation. These risk factors include the presence of gangrene, a high resistance, non-availability of a saphenous vein, and diabetes. All of these risk factors presenting in a single patient would suggest a poor outcome.

On-table arteriography and measurement of peripheral resistance

If the preoperative arteriograms are of good quality and the vessel to be used for the anastomosis is easily seen, then this vessel should be exposed as described below. If the vessels were not easily seen preoperatively, then before the patient is brought to theatre other methods should be used to decide which vessel should be explored, as discussed earlier in this chapter. The chosen vessel, which is often the popliteal trifurcation, should be exposed and an on-table arteriogram done. Whichever vessel is chosen for anastomosis is examined by arteriography before measuring peripheral resistance. The technique for on-table arteriography and measurement of peripheral resistance has already been described in Chapter 2 but will be briefly repeated here.

Having identified the artery to be used, this vessel is exposed as described below. The vessel is opened through an arteriotomy of sufficient size to introduce a silastic cannula (Fig. 13.4). Care must be taken when this is being done otherwise the intima of the vessel can be damaged, particularly if it is calcified. Once the cannula has been inserted (the size will depend on the vessel available), it is attached to a three-way tap (to allow the pressure to be measured) and also to a long connecting tube which can be used to

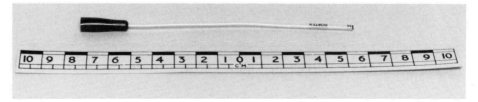

Fig. 13.4
Silastic catheter used for peripheral resistance measurements.

attach it to either an infusion pump or a syringe for arteriography. The cannula can be kept in place by looping a silastic sling around the artery and applying a clip to maintain a seal. An arteriogram is now performed and, while the film is being developed (Fig. 13.5), the peripheral resistance can be measured. This is done by connecting the cannula to a glass syringe fixed to a constant infusion pump (Fig. 13.6) capable of delivering a flow of 100 ml/min. The glass syringe is previously filled with blood taken from the patient's exposed femoral artery. The resistance is measured using the following formula:

Resistance[1] (PRU) =

$$\frac{\text{Arterial pressure} - \text{Venous pressure}}{\text{Flow}}$$

(1 PRU = 1000 mPRU)

Using this system it has been possible to show that, if the resistance is higher than 1400 mPRU, the graft is unlikely to remain patent.[5] The injection of papaverine to increase flow has not helped to improve the accuracy of this test.

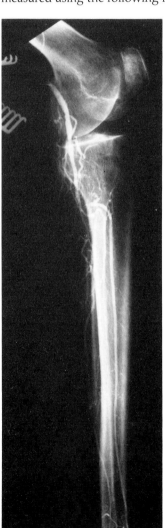

Fig. 13.5
Preoperative on-table angiogram of the popliteal artery showing that the anterior tibial artery is the best vessel to attach the graft to.

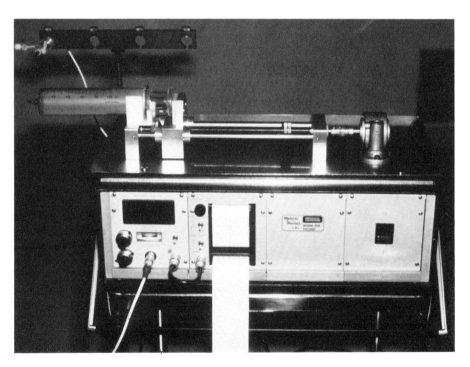

Fig. 13.6
Pump used to inject blood into the potential recipient vessel to measure resistance.

This procedure is a little complicated and may be time consuming and an alternative potentially simpler technique has recently been published using a spring-loaded syringe[9] (Fig. 13.7) (see p. 14).

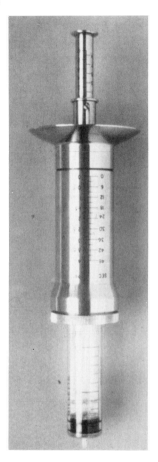

Fig. 13.7
Spring-loaded syringe that can be used to measure peripheral resistance instead of the pump shown in Figure 13.6.

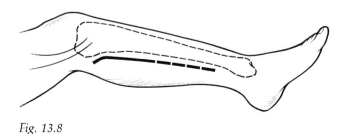

Fig. 13.8

EXPOSURE OF THE POSTERIOR TIBIAL ARTERY AND BYPASS GRAFTING

Before any measurement or arteriography is performed, the artery has, of course, to be exposed. The patient is placed in the prone position with the knee bent to 20°–30°. This position can be maintained by a sandbag behind the knee, or by fixing the foot with a sandbag against the sole. If the precise point of anastomosis is already known from preoperative arteriography, then the vessel can be approached directly. If, however, as is often the case, the level of the distal anastomosis is uncertain (especially if PGR has not been done) the popliteal trifurcation should be exposed as described in Chapter 10 and the vessel followed downwards. An incision is made immediately behind the medial border of the tibia and extended upwards, following the curve of the gastrocnemius muscle backwards (Fig. 13.8). The backward element should be avoided if an amputation is likely, otherwise it will interfere with the flaps if subsequent below-knee amputation is required. This incision can be extended distally as far as is necessary, but initially it should be taken to about halfway down the leg. The long saphenous vein will be immediately anterior to the incision and in thin subjects can usually be seen before the incision is made and safeguarded. If the vessel is not seen, however, it must be carefully looked for and protected. Preoperative mapping with Duplex or venography can help to do this.

Having incised the skin and deep fascia, the medial border of the tibia and the gastrocnemius muscle will be seen. The fascia between the gastrocnemius muscle and the tibia is now divided with scissors and the medial head thereby pushed posteriorly (Fig. 13.9). Having done this, the soleus muscle will be exposed as it curves round towards the tibia. By retracting the medial head of gastrocnemius posteriorly it will be possible to see the popliteal vein covering the artery as they pass beneath the soleus muscle.

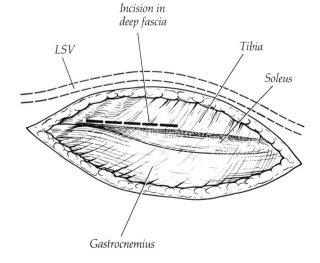

Fig. 13.9

At this point the fascia over the vein should carefully be divided with scissors and the soleus separated by sharp dissection from its attachment to the tibia, thereby exposing the vessel (Fig. 13.10). Sometimes it is necessary to detach the medial head of gastrocnemius from its origin, but this is not usually required. As the dissection passes downwards and the soleus is separated from the tibia by sharp dissection, the popliteal artery and its tributaries will be encountered. Careful dissection with scissors and forceps will allow the popliteal trifurcation and the origins of the anterior tibial, the peroneal and the posterior tibial arteries to be exposed. Throughout this part of their course the arteries are invariably surrounded by the popliteal vein and its branches, which criss-cross either in front of or behind the vessels. These branches need to be controlled and tied before division to expose the various elements of the vessel. An arteriogram should now be performed (Fig. 13.11) using the popliteal artery above the trifurcation in order to obtain a picture. A butterfly needle or, if resistance is being measured, a cannula can be used for this purpose. If this proves impossible, or if there is no lumen, then the posterior tibial artery should be followed downwards to the point where, on pre-operative investigation, a patent vessel is thought to be available. Alternatively, the needle can be inserted where the vessel feels soft—if blood is obtained a reasonable arteriogram is easily obtainable.

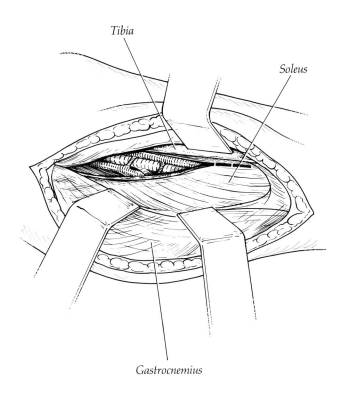

Fig. 13.10

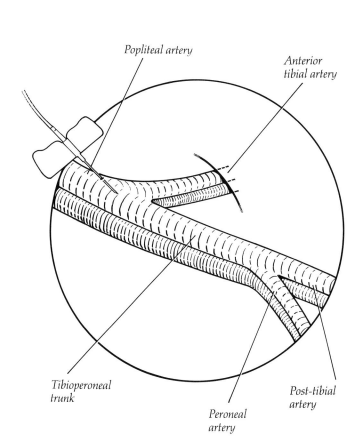

Fig. 13.11

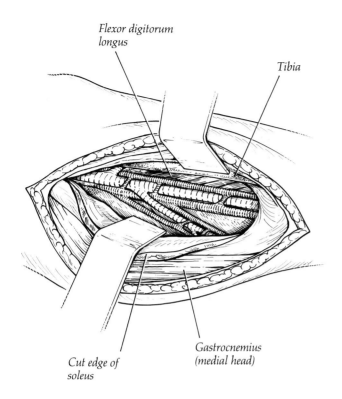

Flexor digitorum longus

Tibia

Cut edge of soleus

Gastrocnemius (medial head)

Fig. 13.12

The posterior tibial artery can be dissected free as far down the leg as necessary, enlarging the skin incision and separating the soleus muscle from the tibia (Fig. 13.12). Slings are placed around the artery, above and below the point where an anastomosis is going to take place (Fig. 13.13). The site for an anastomosis can be as low as the ankle. If it is known that the vessel is patent near to the ankle then dissection can be limited to the ankle area, exposing the vessel directly as it lies behind the tibialis posterior and flexor digitorum longus muscles. In order to expose the vessel in the lower part of the leg, an incision is made immediately behind the tibia to its posterio-medial side (Fig. 13.14), bearing in mind that the artery will eventually pass behind the medial malleolus—be careful to preserve the long saphenous vein although it should by now be anterior to the incision.

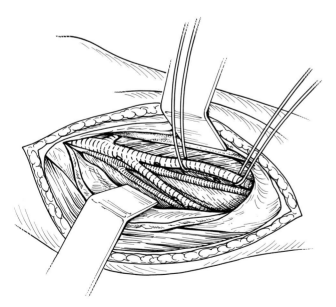

Fig. 13.13

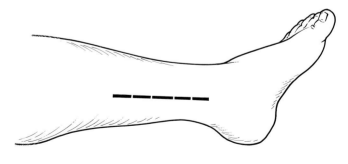

Fig. 13.14

By separating the tibialis posterior and flexor digitorum longus muscles anteriorly and the soleus and gastrocnemius tendons posteriorly the artery and veins will easily be seen lying on the flexor hallucis longus. By careful sharp dissection, the artery is separated from the vein and surrounded by fine silastic slings in the usual way (Fig. 13.15). An arteriogram should now be performed and, if all is well and a decision is taken to proceed, the femoral artery should be exposed in the groin as already described for femoropopliteal and in situ grafting (p. 110). If the long saphenous vein is to be used as an in situ graft, then it should be prepared in exactly the same way as already described using a continuous or inter-mittent incisions. Once the proximal anastomosis has been performed as for in situ graft (p. 145), the distal vein is then sutured carefully to the chosen posterior tibial artery. This is a difficult anastomosis and requires magnification to do properly; a loupe is quite satis-factory for this purpose. Interrupted sutures should be used for the toe of the anastomosis and 7/0 Prolene is best for this procedure, which is described fully on page 148 and briefly summarised in Figures 13.16 to 13.22. Before completing the anastomosis, back bleeding is looked for and adequate forward flow assured by releasing the proximal clamp. A postoperative completion on-table angiogram should be performed before closing the wound. It is important to ensure that the graft does not kink as it passes from the superficial location to join the deeper crural artery. Sometimes it can be kinked by the tendons of the gracilis and semi-tendinosus muscles and if necessary these can be cut, although they should be preserved if possible.

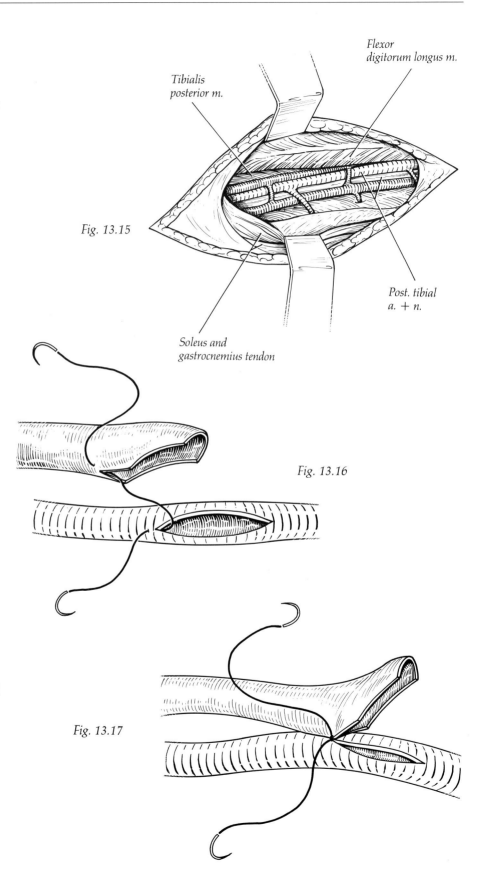

Tibialis posterior m.

Flexor digitorum longus m.

Post. tibial a. + n.

Soleus and gastrocnemius tendon

Fig. 13.15

Fig. 13.16

Fig. 13.17

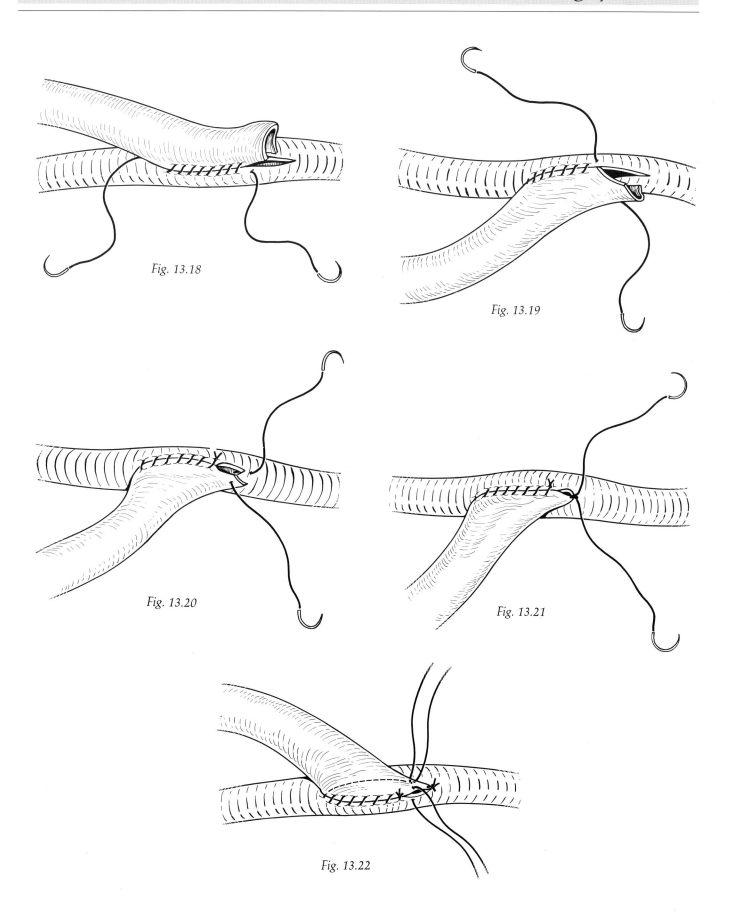

Fig. 13.18

Fig. 13.19

Fig. 13.20

Fig. 13.21

Fig. 13.22

If the long saphenous vein is not available and a decision has been made to use artificial materials, then either human umbilical vein graft or PTFE with external support should be considered. In this event the graft should next be tunnelled in the anatomical position by passing a tunneller from the lower incision proximally alongside the artery, as described on page 133 for femoro-popliteal grafting. In the lower leg the tunnel will pass deep to the gas-trocnemius between its two heads and into the thigh medial to the tendon of the adductor magnus. It may be necessary to do this in two stages (Fig. 13.23). Once the tunneller emerges from the groin wound, the graft is pulled through it with long forceps and, after straightening the limb, an end-to-side anastomosis performed as already described (p. 147). If, for some reason, an anatomical route is not available or is felt to be difficult to negotiate, then the graft can be placed subcutaneously. This is done by passing the tunnelling device from below under the skin until it reaches the knee joint area. At this point the tunneller should be pointed slightly backwards in order to allow a slight curve of no more than 5°–10° across the knee joint. The straight path of the tunneller can then be resumed towards the upper wound. It may be necessary to do this in two stages by making an entry incision at the knee area. A slight curve of the knee prevents kinking when the knee is bent. A subcutaneous route is perfectly acceptable, but it does mean the graft is perhaps exposed to trauma and can be compressed during sleep. It can also ulcerate through the skin and cause problems.

EXPOSURE OF THE PERONEAL ARTERY AND GRAFTING

The peroneal artery is frequently the only vessel left in the critically ischaemic lower leg. The use of this vessel for grafting is controversial and the results are by no means uniform. The vessel can be exposed using either the medial approach, as described for the posterior tibial artery, before it perforates the interosseous membrane midway down the calf, or at the ankle where it lies behind the membrane, which has to be divided to obtain access—often difficult. Thirdly, it can be approached laterally by removing a portion of fibula overlying the chosen site. Generally speaking, the upper two-thirds of the vessel can be exposed through a medial approach, which is the one to be preferred. For this operation the steps are exactly as those described for the exposure of the posterior tibial artery, except of course the peroneal artery lies more deeply. About halfway down the leg the vessel is covered by the flexor hallucis longus and separation of this muscle from the tibia will allow exposure of the peroneal artery (Figs 13.24–13.27). The steps thereafter are exactly the same as those described for femoroposterior tibial bypass grafting. At the ankle the vessel is exposed by first of all isolating the posterior tibial artery, as already described, and then dividing the underlying interosseous membrane longitudinally—the vessel lies immediately underneath it. Access at this point is quite difficult, however, because of the depth of the wound and the limited exposure between the tibia and fibula.

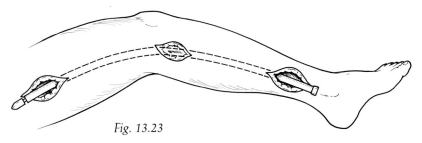

Fig. 13.23

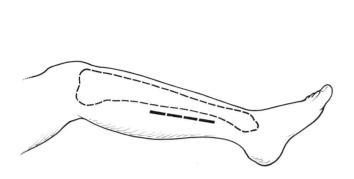

Fig. 13.24

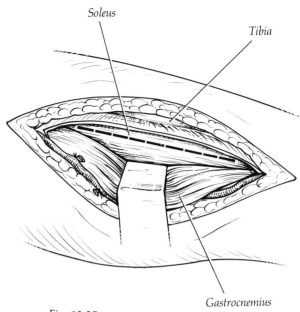

Soleus

Tibia

Gastrocnemius

Fig. 13.25

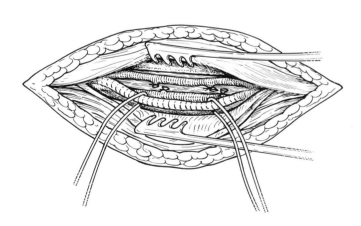

Fig. 13.26

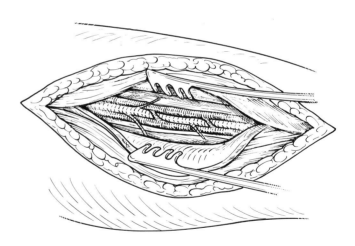

Fig. 13.27

Lateral approach by removing part of the fibula

Some surgeons prefer this approach, but generally it is not necessary as most of the artery can be exposed from a medial incision. An incision is made in the midpart of the leg overlying the fibula, which can be traced upwards by palpation of its lower subcutaneous portion (Fig. 13.28). The incision lies immediately in front of the bulge of muscle caused by the lateral head of gastrocnemius and soleus. The incision is deepened posteriorly through the gastrocnemius and the peroneal muscles until the fibula is seen. Using sharp dissection, the muscles are cleared from the bone until 8–10 cm of it are visible. This portion is now removed using either a Gigli saw (Fig. 13.29) or strong bone-cutting forceps. When encircling the fibula great care needs to be taken to avoid damage to the peroneal artery which lies immediately behind it. After the bone has been excised, the peroneal artery and veins will be seen and can be exposed by sharp dissection with scissors (Fig. 13.30). The artery is then separated from the veins and controlled with fine silastic slings as already described.

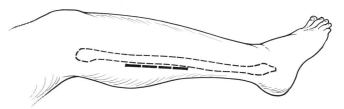

Fig. 13.28

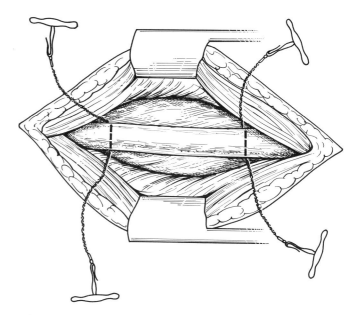

Fig. 13.29

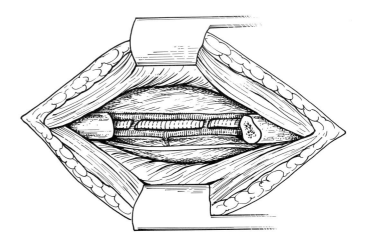

Fig. 13.30

If the long saphenous vein in situ has been used, the operation will proceed as for in situ graft, ensuring that the lower end is long enough to pass through the interosseous membrane (Fig. 13.31). This will necessitate a deepening of the medial wound where the in situ graft is being dissected free and exposure of the membrane by division of the soleus muscle, as previously described for exposure of the posterior tibial artery. A guide to the length of the vein needed can be obtained using a piece of silastic sling passed through the membrane. After division of its lower end and disruption of the valves, as described for the in situ technique on page 140, care must be taken to avoid twisting the vein and ensuring that an adequate window in the membrane has been cut to avoid constricting the graft (Fig. 13.32). The vein is then sewn to the artery end-to-side using continuous 7/0 Prolene, with interrupted sutures to the toe of the anastomosis. A completion angiogram of a femoroperoneal vein graft is shown in Figure 13.33. If an artificial graft such as PTFE or HUVG is being used, a similar route can be employed with the graft in the anatomical position, the lower end passing through the inter-rosseous membrane. However, a simpler technique which avoids a medial incision is to use a subcutaneous route and pass the graft laterally across the thigh, curving gently backwards to join the peroneal artery on the lateral side of the leg (Fig. 13.31). This passage is made with a tunneller as described for a graft to the posterior tibial artery.

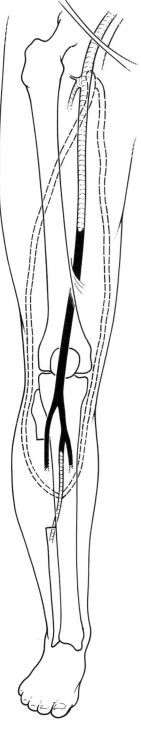

Fig. 13.31

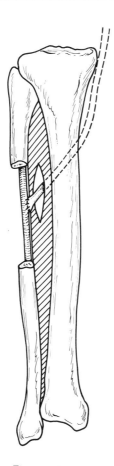

Fig. 13.32

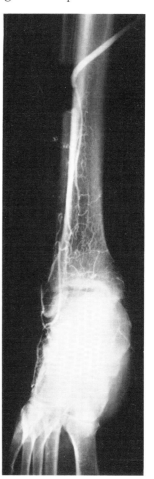

Fig. 13.33
Completion angiogram after femoroperoneal in situ vein graft.

EXPOSURE OF THE ANTERIOR TIBIAL ARTERY AND GRAFTING

An incision is made in the mid-third of the lower leg immediately lateral to the edge of the tibia (Fig. 13.34). The incision is deepened between the tibialis anterior muscle and the extensor digitorum longus. Space is often at a premium in this compartment and the incision should be longer than would normally be required. In particular, the fascial incision should be adequate as the layer of fascia in this area is thick and retraction can otherwise be a problem. Once dissection through the muscle is complete, the artery is easily seen lying on the interosseous membrane (Fig. 13.35). If it cannot be found, then a branch of the artery which can usually be seen easily is followed back to the main vessel. By careful sharp dissection, the artery is separated from its accompanying veins and controlled with fine silastic slings. The graft will take the same route as for the peroneal artery and will depend upon which graft is being used. If the long saphenous vein is being used in situ then the operation will proceed as for in situ vein grafting. The medial incision is deepened after dividing the soleus muscle until the interosseous membrane is seen and felt, as for exposure of the posterior tibial artery in mid calf. An incision is then made through the membrane, of sufficient size to allow the vein to pass through it. The vein is then taken through the hole in the interosseous membrane, which should be above the point at which the anastomosis is being made in order to allow the graft to pass through it obliquely and lie side by side with the anterior tibial artery to which it is being anastomosed. An anastomosis is then constructed as previously described for the posterior tibial artery, using continuous 7/0 Prolene with interrupted sutures at the toe of the anastomosis. If PTFE or HUVG is being used, this route can also be utilised and the graft fed through the interosseous membrane as just described. It may be easier to take the graft laterally passing across the thigh, angling gently backwards and then inserting into the anterior tibial artery. The tunnel is made subcutaneously as before (Fig. 13.31).

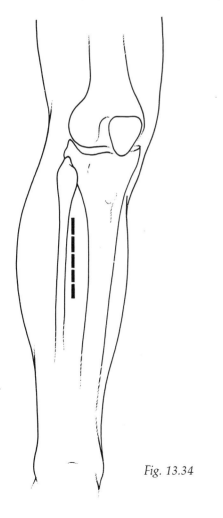

Fig. 13.34

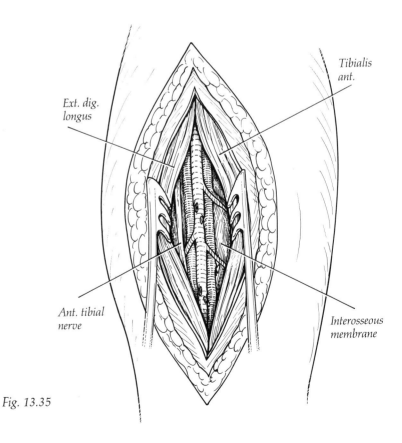

Fig. 13.35

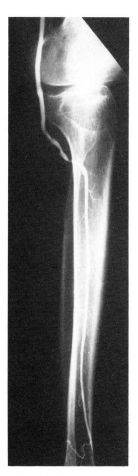

Fig. 13.36
Completion angiogram of a femoroanterior tibial in situ vein graft. There is some stenosis of the anastomosis.

All of these procedures should be checked by completion angiography, and an example of a vein graft to the origin of the anterior tibial artery is shown in Figure 13.36.

The vessel can also be exposed laterally after removing a portion of fibula and incising the interosseous membrane although access is not very good when this approach is used. It can also be exposed medially in the lower part of the leg. A medial incision is made as for exposure of the posterior tibial artery and the vessel approached by incising the interosseous membrane on which it lies.

DECISION POINTS IN THE OPERATION

These operations are difficult and should only be used for limb salvage procedures. The results are not good enough to merit their application to patients with claudication. If the peripheral resistance has been measured and is higher than 1400 mPRU, a primary amputation should be considered. An alternative is to construct an adjunctive arteriovenous fistula, as described later.

SPECIAL PROBLEMS WITH DIFFERENT GRAFTS

If PTFE is being used it is vital that the opening in the artery should be exactly equal to that in the graft. This material does not stretch and if it is too short or too long narrowing of the anastomosis will occur and lead to thrombosis. Because of possible kinking with knee movements, an externally supported prosthesis is now available for use below the knee. If this graft is used, the external support should be peeled back from the area of the anastomosis. If human umbilical vein is used then the distal anastomosis can be quite difficult because the graft wall is very thick; the newer thin-walled varieties are easier to use. Generally speaking, the graft can be sewn on fairly easily, but great care needs to be taken with the toe of the graft where interrupted sutures should be inserted and tied after they have all been placed (Figs 13.37 and 13.38). The other problem with umbilical vein graft is that it is not possible to readjust its position once the tunneller has been removed. It will not slide in the tunnel made for it and attempts to pull it up or down will simply disrupt the graft and lead to thrombosis. For this reason it is vital that, before the tunneller is

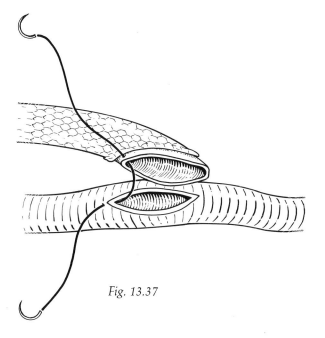

Fig. 13.37

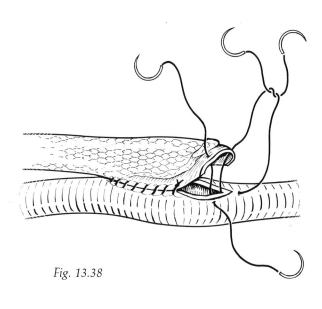

Fig. 13.38

removed, its position and length is confirmed to be that required. For the lower anastomosis it is not essential to include the net in the anastomosis—this can be tacked to the artery with separate sutures later (Fig. 13.39).

Because of the difficulties sometimes experienced with the anastomosis between human umbilical vein and small distal arteries, it is possible to obtain a piece of vein from some part of the body—either a piece of long saphenous vein at the ankle or the cephalic vein from the arm—and to use this as a composite graft (Fig. 13.40). In this procedure the piece of vein, usually no more than 2 or 3 cm in length, is stitched end-to-end with umbilical vein graft, allowing the distal anastomosis with a fine often calcified tibial vessel to be made between the artery and a piece of thin vein. Unfortunately, although composite grafts have now been used intermittently, the change in compliance between the two vessels and between the vein and the artery tend to lead to worse results and this procedure is not generally recommended.

Vein cuff to PTFE grafts

The insertion of PTFE grafts to distal ankle vessels often produces poor results.[10,11] This can be improved to some extent by the attachment of a collar of vein to the recipient artery to intervene between the PTFE and the vessel. This is done by removing a small piece of vein from the arm or the leg, opening it longitudinally (Fig. 13.41) and stitching it to the arteriotomy (Fig. 13.42), using a continuous suture, thereby providing the cuff to which the PTFE is sutured in an end-to-side fashion (Figs 13.43 and 13.44). This approach allows a reasonable one-year graft patency rate which may be sufficient to allow lesions of the foot to heal.[12] An alternative approach is to use a patch of vein to complete one side of the anastomosis, as described by Taylor, which can also produce good results.[13]

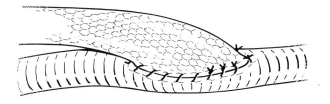

Fig. 13.39

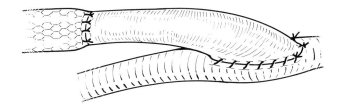

Fig. 13.40

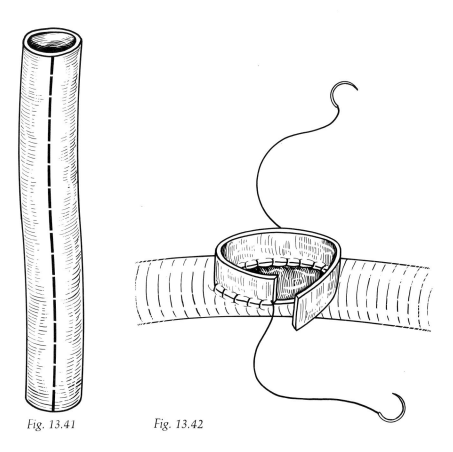

Fig. 13.41   Fig. 13.42

Complications of femorocrural grafting

The main complication of this procedure is early occlusion of the graft. If this occurs in the first 24–48 hours or during the hospital stay, the patient should be taken to theatre and the graft re-explored to exclude a technical problem. The best plan is to open both top and bottom wounds, heparinise the patient and undo one side of the lower anastomosis. This will allow direct access to the area most likely to be causing a problem. A Fogarty catheter can then be passed distally and proximally until flow is re-established. Once the anastomosis has been cleared, a further on-table angiogram on completion is essential. Another complication that can occur with subcutaneously placed artificial grafts is infection and erosion of the graft through the skin. This complication usually occurs days or weeks after the procedure and frequently means that the graft has to be removed with consequent limb loss. Persistent arteriovenous (AV) fistulae can occur with the in situ technique and can cause skin necrosis necessitating ligation of the communication.

RESULTS

Results vary depending upon the publication but are generally relatively poor compared with proximal lesions. They do, however, depend very much on the outflow available in the limb and the foot distal to the anastomosis. Saphenous vein sutured in situ (three-year patency 80%) tends to do better than artificial grafts (three-year patency 35%). If the long saphenous vein is not available, then either a human umbilical vein graft or PTFE can be used, but inferior results have to be expected.[10, 11] There is no doubt that limb salvage and patency rates depend very much on the outflow.[4] Patients who have more than one outflow vessel available do better than those with a single artery, who in turn do better than those with stenosed run-off vessels.

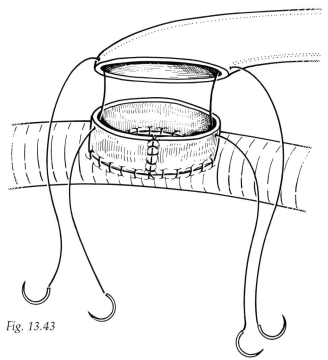

Fig. 13.43

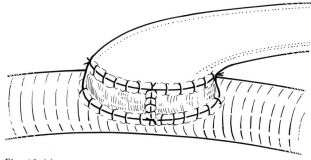

Fig. 13.44

ARTERIOVENOUS FISTULAE AND MULTIPLE ANASTOMOSES

In these cases, if the resistance in the outflow vessels is very high as described on page 13, or if the arterial arcades in the foot are poor and success is thought to be unlikely, various methods of improving results have been suggested. The first is the creation of an arteriovenous fistula[14] and the second is multiple separate anastomoses to the distal foot vessels.

Arteriovenous fistula

The artery chosen for the anastomosis will have been exposed in one of the ways already described along with its accompanying veins. The vein and artery are separately controlled with fine silastic slings and the larger of the two accompanying veins selected for the anastomosis (Fig. 13.45). A loupe is usually required for this procedure. Using a scalpel and right-angled arterial scissors, a longitudinal incision is made in the artery and vein side by side. The exact length of the two openings remains controversial. They can be of exactly the same length (Fig. 13.46), or the incision in the vein can be approximately one-third that of the artery. This modification makes the anastomosis easier and theoretically at least reduces the amount of blood passing up the vein as a steal. Using double-ended 7/0 or 8/0 Prolene sutures, the vessels are sewn together as in Figure 13.47, the needle passing from the inside to the outside of the vein and artery and tied externally.

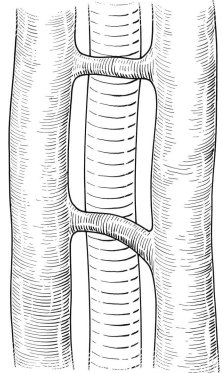

Fig. 13.45

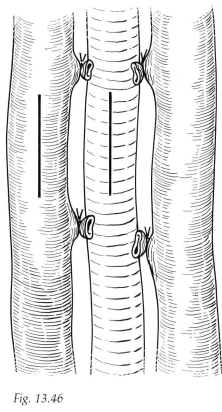

Fig. 13.46

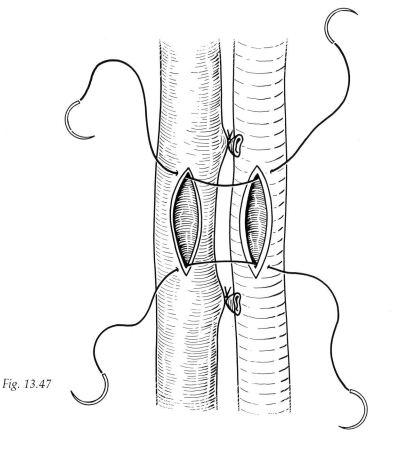

Fig. 13.47

Using one of the two sutures of what will become the toe (distal) end of the anastomosis the posterior wall is now sutured (Fig. 13.48). When the posterior wall has been completed, the needle is passed to the outside and the suture is tied to one of the two sutures at the heel end of the anastomosis. The chosen graft is next cut to the exact size of the common arteriovenous osteum and anastomosed as in Figure 13.49 using the existing two sutures at the heel of the anastomosis.

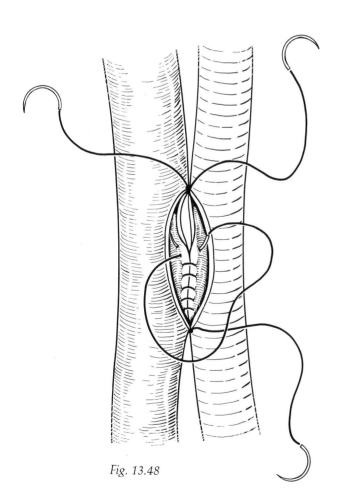

Fig. 13.48

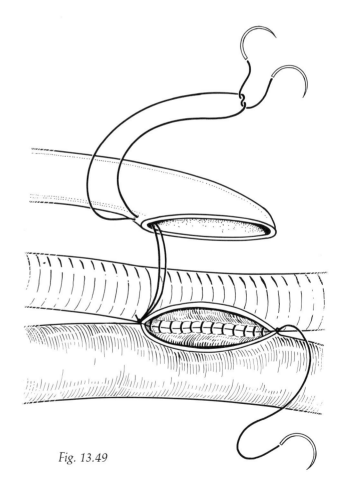

Fig. 13.49

Each stitch is passed in turn from the outside to the inside of the graft and the inside to the outside of the artery. The graft is sutured to the common osteum, completing the suture line as in Figure 13.50 and stopping on each side 3–4 mm from the toe. Each stitch is then tied in this position. The remaining part of the anastomosis is now completed with interrupted sutures (Fig. 13.50). Generally speaking, approximately five of these are required. They are tied individually once they have all been placed (Fig. 13.51) after proximal and retrograde bleeding has first of all been confirmed. When the clamps are released there should be a palpable thrill at the anastomosis and the veins should be seen to pulsate both proximally and possibly distally. Distal pulsation may not travel very far, especially if a valve is present in the vein.

This particular configuration for the anastomosis may not offer the best haemodynamic advantages. Experimental work has suggested that a fistula placed proximal to the anastomosis between the graft and the artery may be a significantly better haemodynamic arrangement[15] but this remains to be tested in patients (Fig. 13.52). Some swelling of the foot may occur after this procedure, but this soon passes when the patient mobilises. Apart from this there are no other significant problems. Results have, however, been mixed. Dardik has suggested that these patients do well,[14] but other authors have suggested that the addition of an AV fistula to these anastomoses makes no difference to the outcome.[16] It is likely that they might be useful in selected cases, particularly if the long saphenous vein is used as the graft material.

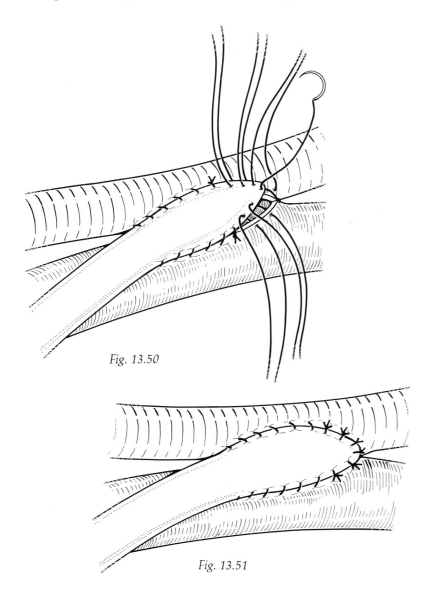

Fig. 13.50

Fig. 13.51

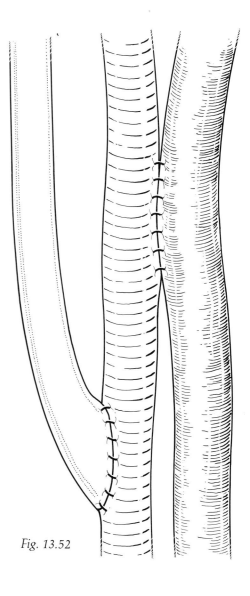

Fig. 13.52

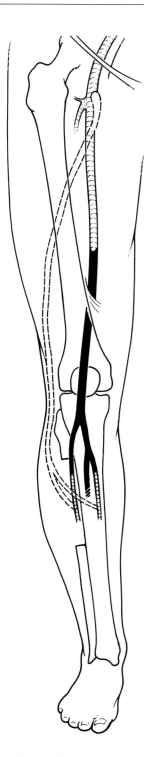

Multiple anastomoses

If more than one outflow vessel is available and if, as is usually the case, the long saphenous vein has a number of branches, then separate anastomoses can be constructed between the vein and the two arteries using separate incisions to expose the vessels as already described. One branch can be anastomosed, for example to the posterior tibial artery near to or at the ankle. A second branch can be anastomosed to the anterior tibial artery near to the ankle after passing the graft through the interosseous membrane, or allowing it to pass over the front of the tibia: both work equally well. Using this technique can be very successful, but its use obviously depends on the availability of more than one outflow vessel. Magnification is, of course, required (Fig. 13.53).

COMPLICATIONS OF AN ADJUNCTIVE AV FISTULA

These are relatively few and amount mainly to graft occlusion in these high-risk cases. This may, however, be followed by the need for a higher amputation than would otherwise have been necessary, particularly if graft sepsis occurs with artificial materials. Generally speaking, the addition of an arterio-venous fistula does not cause any haemo-dynamic problems as the deep veins are involved in the anastomosis.

Fig. 13.53

ANASTOMOSES TO THE FOOT VESSELS

It is becoming clear that a number of patients with rest pain have patent popliteal arteries with occlusion of most of the intervening crural vessels and patent anterior or posterior tibial arteries or their branches in the foot. In this situation, a vein graft either in situ or reversed between a patent popliteal artery and the patent foot vessels (Fig. 13.54) can produce good results for limb salvage.[17] Adequate distal angiography is essential if these procedures are to be undertaken. The anterior tibial artery is exposed through a vertical or curved incision (Fig. 13.55). The vessel lies immediately under the skin in the midline of the foot and is easily exposed by superficial dissection. An appropriate segment is isolated between silastic slings. The long saphenous vein is dissected through a separate incision (Fig. 13.56) and swung across to meet the artery (Fig. 13.57)—the two incisions can sometimes be continuous. It is important in this area to use the end-to-side technique with a loupe for magnification purposes and interrupted 7 or 8/0 sutures (Fig. 13.58). If a reversed vein graft is used, the tunnel between the patent popliteal artery and the tibial vessel can be superficial, with the lower end of the vein curving round the lower end of the tibia. If the patent artery is more distal, i.e. the deep branch of the dorsalis pedis, this can be approached by a vertical incision between the first and second metatarsal bones with lateral retraction of the extensor hallucis brevis muscle (Fig. 13.59). Resection of part of the second metatarsal allows even better access to the deep plantar arch for a distal anastomosis (Fig. 13.60). Once again the saphenous vein is mobilised as far distally as possible and swung laterally to meet the artery where the anastomosis is required.

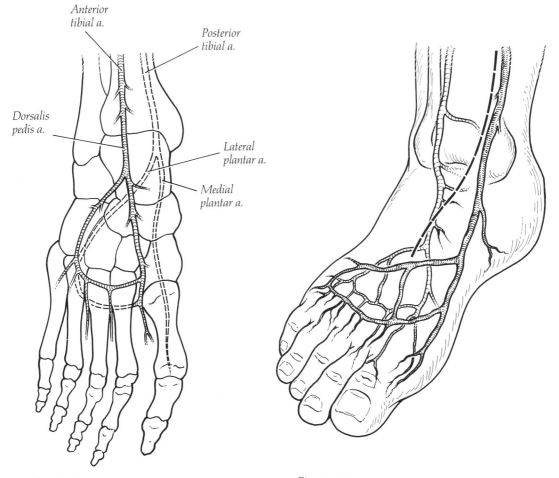

Anterior tibial a.

Posterior tibial a.

Dorsalis pedis a.

Lateral plantar a.

Medial plantar a.

Fig. 13.54

Fig. 13.55

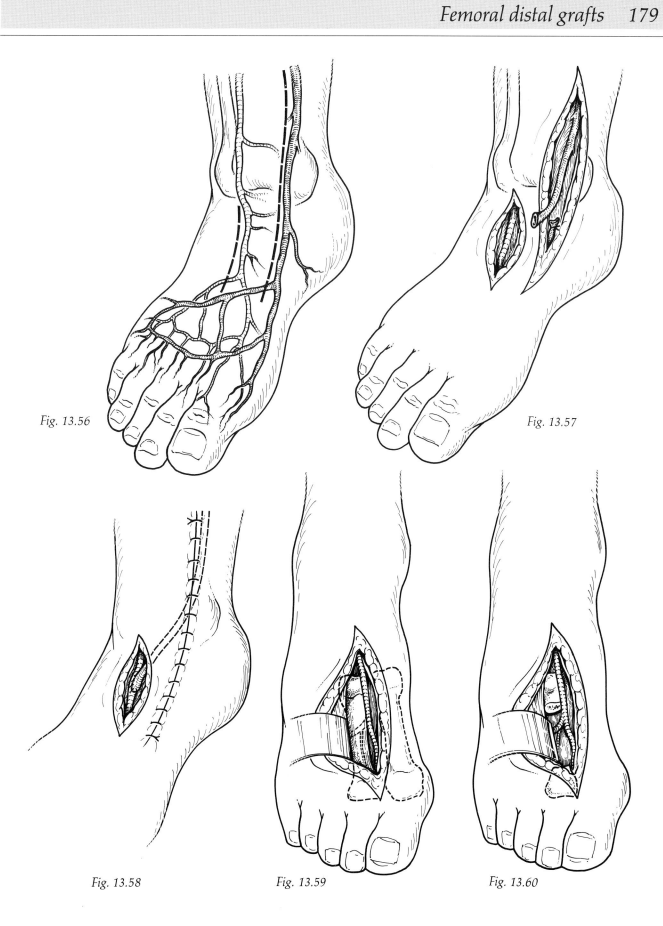

Fig. 13.56

Fig. 13.57

Fig. 13.58

Fig. 13.59

Fig. 13.60

Posterior tibial artery

This vessel is often patent behind the medial malleolus where it can be approached relatively easily as it lies behind the retinaculum (Fig. 13.61). The long saphenous vein is again mobilised through an incision over it and swung backwards to allow end-to-side anastomosis to the posterior tibial artery (Fig. 13.62). Sometimes the posterior tibial artery needs to be approached more deeply after it has divided into the medial and lateral plantar arteries. The incision, if taken more distally, allows access to both branches and the lateral or medial branch might be the artery of choice for the anastomosis (Fig. 13.63)—this will depend upon the arteriogram.

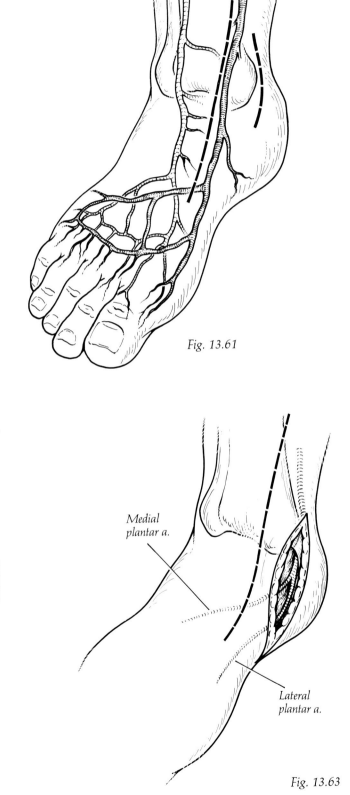

Fig. 13.61

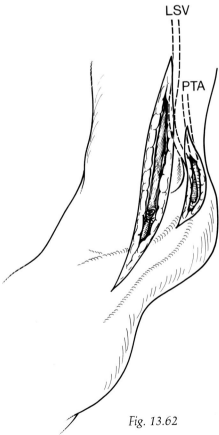

LSV

PTA

Fig. 13.62

Medial plantar a.

Lateral plantar a.

Fig. 13.63

Peroneal artery

This vessel will usually be available higher up, but can be approached near the ankle, again by an incision over the lateral part of the leg immediately in front of the fibula (Fig. 13.64). At this point the vessel can be exposed, but access is difficult. The long saphenous vein is mobilised through a separate incision, sufficient length being mobilised to allow its easy apposition to the peroneal artery (Fig. 13.65).

Technical improvements have meant that more distal anastomoses have become possible, particularly to the crural and foot vessels. However, it should be remembered that results can be poor and, in a patient with a relatively small chance of success, technical innovations must not be allowed to override common sense—in some situations an amputation might be the best choice. For this reason, it is important that surgeons involved in these areas develop the ability and the will to make objective measurements of likely outcome before proceeding to complicated bypass operations.

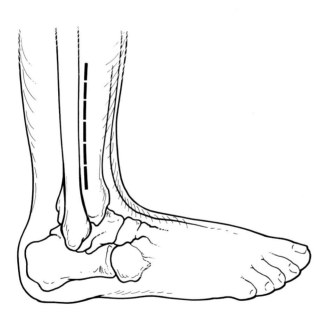

Fig. 13.64

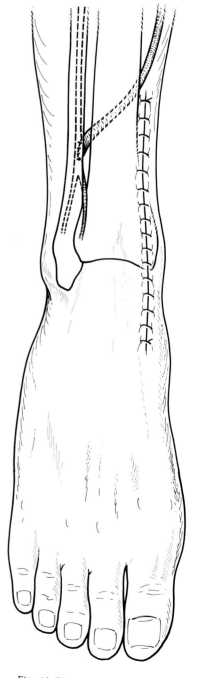

Fig. 13.65

REFERENCES

1 Bell P R F 1985 Are distal vascular procedures worthwhile? British Journal of Surgery 75: 335
2 European consensus on critical limb ischaemia 1989 Lancet 1: 737
3 Beard J D, Scott D J A, Evans M, Skidmore R, Horrocks M 1988 Pulse generated run-off—a new method of determining calf vessel patency. British Journal of Surgery 75: 361–363
4 Parvin S D, Evans D H, Bell P R F 1985 Peripheral resistance measurement in the assessment of severe peripheral vascular disease. British Journal of Surgery 72: 751–753
5 Bagi P, Schroder T, Silleson H, Lorentzen J E 1989 Real time B mode mapping of the greater saphenous vein. European Journal of Vascular Surgery 3: 103–107
6 Andros G, Harris R W, Dulawa L B, Oblath R W, Salles-Cunha S X 1989 In: Greenhalgh R (ed) Vascular surgical techniques—an atlas. Saunders, London, pp 235–242
7 Dardik H, Kahn M, Dardik I, Sussman B, Ibrahim I M 1987 Influence of failed vascular bypass procedures on conversion of below-knee to above-knee amputation levels. Surgery 91: 64–69
8 Ascer E, Veith F J, Morin L et al 1984 Quantitative assessment of outflow resistance in lower extremity arterial reconstruction. Journal of Surgical Research 37: 8–15
9 Beard J D, Scott D J A, Evans M, Skidmore R, Horrocks M 1988 A simple method of measuring peripheral resistance. In: Price, Evans (eds) Blood flow measurement in clinical diagnosis. Conference proceedings, Biological Engineering Society pp 64–68

10 Klimach O, Underwood C J, Charlesworth D 1984 Femoropopliteal bypass with Goretex prosthesis—a long-term follow up. British Journal of Surgery 71: 821–824
11 Rutherford R B, Jones D N, Bergentz S E et al 1988 Factors affecting the patency of infrainguinal bypass. Journal of Vascular Surgery 8: 237–246
12 Miller J H, Foreman R K, Ferguson L, Faris I 1984 Interposition vein cuff for anastomosis of prosthesis to small artery. Australian and New Zealand Journal of Surgery 54: 283–286
13 Taylor R S, McFarland R J, Cox M I 1987 An investigation into the causes of failure of PTFE grafts. European Journal of Vascular Surgery 1(5): 327–335
14 Dardik H, Sussman B, Ibrahim M 1983 Distal arteriovenous fistula as an adjunct to maintaining arterial and graft patency for limb salvage. Surgery 94: 478–482
15 Parvin S D, Bentley S, Asher M J, Prytherch D R, Evans D H, Bell P R F 1984 Haemodynamics of the adjunctive arteriovenous fistula in femorodistal bypass grafting—an experimental study. British Journal of Surgery 71: 502–506
16 Harris P L, Campbell H 1983 Adjuvant distal arteriovenous shunt with femorotibial bypass for critical ischaemia. British Journal of Surgery 70: 377–380
17 Ascer E, Veith F J, Gupta S K 1988 Bypasses to plantar arteries and other tibial branches: an extended approach to limb salvage. Journal of Vascular Surgery 8: 434–442

Chapter 14

Future prospects

This book is designed to try and help those involved with infrainguinal bypass grafts to gain a successful outcome. The reader will by now have gathered that these techniques can be difficult and, in order to gain success, attention to detail is essential.

What does the future hold? It will, I am sure, become much more common to place grafts more distally in the leg in order to save the limbs of older patients, particularly as the population ages and the problem of vascular disease increases. There is no doubt that saphenous vein provides the best result unless a prosthesis can be produced which is usable with small crural vessels. Many patients who are currently considered inoperable will undoubtedly become operable in future as microsurgical techniques become more widespread. It is possible that the newer thrombolytic agents will also allow the run-off vessels to be cleared of thrombus and then revascularised. The use of on-table procedures such as atherectomy and intraoperative angioplasty, with or without laser assistance, in small vessels remains largely unused and there will be a big increase in the use of such techniques in the future. Any trainee vascular surgeon should make himself thoroughly conversant with all of these techniques as he may be called upon to use them in the future.